ALL
ABOUT
VITAMINS
AND
MINERALS

THE NO NONSENSE LIBRARY

NO NONSENSE HEALTH GUIDES

Women's Health and Fitness
A Diet for Lifetime Health
A Guide to Exercise and Fitness Equipment
How to Tone and Trim Your Trouble Spots
Stretch for Health
Unstress Your Life
Calories, Carbohydrates and Sodium
Permanent Weight Loss
Your Emotional Health and Well-Being
Reducing Cholesterol

NO NONSENSE FINANCIAL GUIDES

NO NONSENSE REAL ESTATE GUIDES

NO NONSENSE LEGAL GUIDES

NO NONSENSE CAREER GUIDES

NO NONSENSE SUCCESS GUIDES

NO NONSENSE COOKING GUIDES

NO NONSENSE WINE GUIDES

NO NONSENSE PARENTING GUIDES

NO NONSENSE STUDENT GUIDES

NO NONSENSE HEALTH GUIDE®

ALL ABOUT VITAMINS AND MINERALS

Key Nutrients for Optimum Health

By the Editors of *PREVENTION*® Magazine

Longmeadow Press

Notice

This book is intended as a reference volume only, not as a medical manual or guide to self-treatment. It is not intended as a substitute for the medical advice of physicians. The reader should regularly consult a physician in general, and particularly for any symptoms. If you suspect that you have a medical problem, we urge you to seek competent medical help. Keep in mind that exercise and nutritional needs vary from person to person, depending on age, sex, health status and individual variations. The information here is intended to help you make informed decisions about your health, not as a substitute for any treatment that may have been prescribed by your doctor.

All about Vitamins and Minerals

Copyright ©1989 Rodale Press, Inc. All Rights Reserved.

Published January 1989 by Longmeadow Press, 201 High Ridge Road, Stamford, CT 06904. No part of this book may be reproduced or used in any form or by any means, electronic or mechanical, including photocopying, recording, or by any information storage and retrieval system, without permission in writing from the publisher.

Library of Congress Cataloging-in-Publication Data

All about vitamins and minerals.

(No nonsense health guide)
  1. Nutrition—Popular works.   2. Vitamins—Health aspects.
3. Minerals in the body.
I. Prevention magazine.   II. Title.   III. Series.
RA784.A425   1989   613.2'8   88-26861
ISBN 0-681-40715-8 paperback

Compiled and edited by Marcia Holman and Jane Sherman

Book design by Acey Lee
Cover illustration by Jean Gardner

Photographs by Carl Doney p. 14; John P. Hamel pp. 19, 73; Donna M. Hornberger p. 51; Margaret Skrovanek p. 68; Rodale Press Photography Department pp. 2, 40, 57, 85.

No Nonsense Health Guide is a trademark controlled by Longmeadow Press.

2 4 6 8 10 9 7 5 3   paperback

Contents

We're Getting Smarter about Nutrition

Can the right dose of vitamins or minerals cure disease? Can good nutrition head off health problems and extend your life? Can diet affect the mind as well as the body? Is it necessary to take supplements to stay healthy?

Scientists have been studying these and other questions about nutrition for many years, and the amount of data they have accumulated is considerable. But they're not nearly finished with the search for information: New evidence on the importance of vitamins and minerals is appearing constantly.

Some of this ongoing research is showing that many Americans are increasingly concerned about what's in the 1,500 pounds of food we eat every year. We're eating fewer frankfurters and less luncheon meat, sugar, candy, oils and fats. We're eating more chicken, cheese, dark green vegetables and citrus fruits.

This concern is certainly a step in the right direction. Although clear-cut deficiency conditions like scurvy and beriberi are mostly a thing of the past in this country, it is possible to be lacking in one or more essential nutrients—a lack that may compromise good health. According to some experts, however, most people still have a way to go in understanding nutrition. We may not know how to pick the most nutritious fresh foods and how to read and understand label information on packaged items. We may not realize that certain eating patterns and life-styles may be sabotaging good nutrition, or, if we do, we may not know how to improve the situation.

All about Vitamins and Minerals is designed to help fill the nutritional information gap. It's a quick guide to the nutrients that help us stay healthy and feel great. It explains which vitamins and minerals are vital for boosting energy levels, maintaining bone strength and staying mentally alert. There are lists of the best food sources of many nutrients, and ways to make the most of supplements. All in all, the information provided here should make our goals of better nutrition and better health a little easier to attain.

Spotting Your Nutritional Deficiencies

Food is good medicine. Sure, there's the comfort Mom's chicken soup brings to a fever-worn body, and the warmth of Thanksgiving dinner with the whole family taking part. But we're talking about something more specific: health problems that can be caused by missing out on certain nutrients. And often, alleviating the problem is as easy as putting the right stuff on your plate. Here's a head-to-toe rundown of conditions that can sometimes be traced to disorders in the diet, and the foods that can put things right.

Your Head

A lack of proper nutrition can show up in problems with your vision and the health of your mouth.

Night blindness.   "An early sign of vitamin A deficiency is trouble adapting to darkness," says John Smith, Ph.D., associate professor of nutrition at Pennsylvania State University.

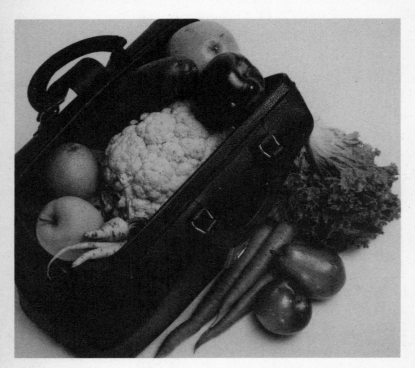

You might be skeptical if your doctor's black bag were filled with fruits and vegetables instead of a stethoscope and pills. The truth is, though, that nutritious food is good medicine and a means to prevent a number of health problems.

"Normally, the human eye can adapt to reduced lighting in less than 1 minute," Dr. Smith explains. "A person whose eyes take 15 to 20 minutes to adapt is said to have night blindness."

Vitamin A supplementation can improve poor night vision caused by a deficiency. "All it takes is to get back up to the Recommended Dietary Allowance (RDA) of 5,000 international units (I.U.), then maintain that RDA through adequate intake of vitamin A in the diet," says Dr. Smith. Good food sources of vitamin A include sweet potatoes, carrots, spinach, cantaloupe, broccoli, winter squash and apricots.

Inflamed gums.   When the body's vitamin C levels near depletion, signs of scurvy, such as gum inflammation and bleeding, begin to show up.

"While this isn't common in the general population, elderly people who live alone and alcoholics are quite susceptible because they tend to have very poor diets," says Jerry Rivers, Ph.D., professor emeritus of nutrition at Cornell University. The deficiency can be corrected in just a few weeks with 200 to 300 milligrams of vitamin C a day, given in three divided doses, Dr. Rivers says.

Vitamin C deficiency may also play a role in periodontal disease, infection caused by residual food, bacteria and tartar that collect in the spaces between the gums and teeth. This condition weakens gums and loosens teeth, and it is the major cause of tooth loss after the age of 35.

While poor nutrition doesn't cause the condition, some researchers believe a deficiency of vitamin C makes it more difficult for the mouth to resist some types of infection.

You can get more vitamin C in your diet by eating citrus fruits, sweet peppers, broccoli, cauliflower, tomatoes, potatoes, peas, melon and strawberries.

Your Midsection

Breathing problems, stooped posture, dry skin and easy bruising are among other signs that something may be amiss in your diet.

Asthma.   In a study by the U.S. Department of Agriculture, researchers noted that 15 asthma patients had significantly lower levels of B_6 than did 16 people without asthma. When given supplements of the vitamin, all of the asthmatic subjects reported "a dramatic decrease in frequency and severity of wheezing or asthmatic attacks while taking the supplement."

Further studies are under way with larger groups of asthma sufferers. In the meantime, the researchers note the 100-milligram doses given during the trial should be used only under medical supervision, as high levels of B_6 may result in nerve damage.

You can safely maintain adequate levels of vitamin B_6 by eating whole grain products, nuts, bananas, poultry and fish.

Poor posture.   An extremely rounded upper back in an elderly person may be a symptom of advanced osteoporosis. When the bones of the spine weaken, they can get squashed, resulting in compression fractures. Osteoporosis doesn't happen overnight. In fact, people with osteoporosis may have been calcium deficient since early adulthood.

Doctors sometimes prescribe large doses of calcium, vitamin D, fluoride and estrogen to improve bone mass, but this treatment is not always effective. The best medicine for osteoporosis is prevention—making sure you get plenty of calcium, vitamin D and exercise.

The best source of calcium is dairy products. Canned fish (bones included) are also a good source, as are broccoli, collards and kale. Fish, fish-liver oils, fortified milk and a bit of sunshine are the best sources of vitamin D.

Dry, rough skin.   This can be an early sign of vitamin A deficiency. The condition, which is known as folliculosis, occurs when small bumps near the base of the hair follicles become hardened.

Broken capillaries.   Vitamin C deficiency can weaken the membranes that line the capillaries, or tiny blood vessels. Where they burst, purplish "bruises" may appear. It's a common problem in people with rheumatoid arthritis. Doctors in England found that vitamin C supplements reduced that bruising. The inflammation that characterizes arthritis tends to deplete vitamin C, and some anti-arthritis drugs interfere with vitamin C metabolism, they say.

Your Lower Body

Inadequate nutrition may also contribute to digestive problems, infertility and muscle cramps.

Constipation and diverticulosis.   Constipation is a frequent hassle for an estimated one out of every eight Americans. What's at the bottom of the problem? "More than any other factor, faulty diet. Specifically, not enough fiber," says James Boylan, M.D., a gastroenterologist from Bethlehem, Pennsylvania. There's some evidence that a low-fiber diet can also contribute to diverticulosis, a condition in which pouches bulge out from the intestines. If the pouches become inflamed (diverticulitis), a person may suffer fever, cramps, constipation and diarrhea. Diverticulosis is common in the elderly, who often choose soft, easy-to-chew foods low in fiber.

Most of us eat only about 10 to 20 grams of dietary fiber a day. Many doctors now recommend 25 to 35 grams a day. Adding more whole grain breads, bran cereals, and fruits and vegetables to your diet will boost your fiber intake and help prevent constipation and possibly diverticulosis.

Infertility.   If one specialist's guess is correct, vitamin C deficiency could be behind as many as 15 percent of the cases of infertility today.

"Sperm agglutination, or clumping, can develop when the body is low in vitamin C," says Earl B. Dawson, Ph.D., associate professor of obstetrics and gynecology at the University of Texas Medical School at Galveston. When sperm clump together, they become less mobile, making it harder for them to travel up the vaginal canal.

Recently, Dr. Dawson and his colleagues gave supplemental vitamin C to men with fertility problems who also had sperm agglutination. After just one week on 1,000-milligram-a-day supplements, the agglutination was reduced substantially. The researchers also saw a dramatic increase in the number of live sperm. No side effects were reported from the high dosage, either.

The second step in the study reduced the vitamin C to 200 milligrams. The same beneficial effects were seen.

"The possibility of sperm impairment from a vitamin C deficiency is certainly something that's worth discussing with a doctor if a couple is having difficulty conceiving," says Dr. Dawson.

Leg cramps.   Calcium, potassium or magnesium deficiency may be what's causing your muscles to kink up. Mineral imbalances aren't very common, so it's a good idea to check with a doctor if you suspect one. At risk are people taking diuretics or steroids, heavy drinkers, pregnant women and older people who may not be eating well.

Magnesium is abundant in beans, nuts, whole wheat products, soy products, bananas and potatoes. Potassium is also found in bananas and potatoes, as well as in raisins, orange juice, fish, tomatoes and milk.

Note: There may be several causes for the conditions discussed in this chapter. A nutritional deficiency is just one possibility. To be sure you're not overlooking a potentially serious condition, consult your doctor before taking action.

What You Should Know about Vitamin Tests

Can medical tests tell you whether you have a vitamin or mineral deficiency—or excess? Is such information really useful to you and your doctor? And will the tests end up costing you more than they're worth?

The answers, as testing experts point out, are yes, maybe and sometimes.

Nowadays, doctors can indeed order laboratory tests for most vitamins and minerals (although medical labs are not equally equipped to assess nutrient levels). Usually your physician gets a blood or urine sample from you and sends it to the lab with instructions to measure the amount of certain nutrients in the sample. The test results may or may not reflect your intake of nutrients but will, in most cases, indicate whether you have high or low levels in your system.

The usefulness of such testing depends, in part, on how widespread vitamin and mineral deficiencies really are. Classic deficiencies —those with unmistakable symptoms, like scurvy and beriberi—are few and far between. Other evidence, however, suggests that milder deficiencies may be more prevalent than people think. (See the table, A Guide to Deficiency Symptoms, on pages 8 and 9.)

A Useful Tool—or a Waste of Time?

One of the researchers who has helped uncover such nutritional deficits is Myron Brin, Ph.D., former adjunct professor at both Columbia Medical School and Cornell Medical School. "We have to be aware," he says, "that national nutritional studies like the Ten-State Survey, the Household Food Consumption Survey and the Health and Nutrition Examination Survey demonstrated that there are many population groups who consume appreciably below Recommended Dietary Allowance (RDA) levels for vitamins A, C and B_6, folate and other nutrients. Such biochemical inadequacy without classic deficiency symptoms is called marginal deficiency—a condition often marked by vague signs like irritability, insomnia and reduced appetite. It's this type of deficiency that nutrient tests can help detect."

But if a doctor suspects that a patient has a deficiency, why can't he forgo nutrient testing and simply prescribe the missing nutrient and see if the symptoms disappear?

He can and often does.

"This technique is called a therapeutic trial," Dr. Brin says. "In some cases, it may be cheaper than nutrient testing. As long as physicians know precisely what symptoms are associated with the deficiency, they can easily assess the effects of the prescribed supplements. If symptoms disappear in about three months, that's evidence that the patient may have lacked the nutrients."

There's more to nutrient testing, however, than just spotting nutritional deficits. Doctors sometimes use it to help confirm the presence of serious medical conditions that may have little or nothing to do with deficiencies. Calcium tests, for example, can help doctors diagnose bone disorders and problems of the parathyroid gland. Magnesium tests can help them detect systemic poisoning, including drug abuse. And the vitamin E test helps them pinpoint the cause of anemia in infants.

None of which means that doctors find nutrient tests as useful as old standbys like routine urinalysis and the complete blood count (the most frequently performed lab test). The majority of physicians use

(continued on page 10)

A Guide to Deficiency Symptoms

Nutrient	Possible Deficiency Symptoms*	RDA for Adults (age 23–50)
Vitamin A	Night blindness; abnormal dryness of the eyeballs; dry, rough, itchy skin; susceptibility to respiratory infection	5,000 I.U. (men) 4,000 I.U. (women)
Thiamine (B_1)	Confusion; weakness of eye muscles; loss of appetite; uncoordinated walk; poor memory; inability to concentrate	1.4 mg. (men) 1.0 mg. (women)
Riboflavin (B_2)	Discolored tongue; anemia; cracks at corners of mouth; scaly skin; burning, itchy eyes	1.6 mg. (men) 1.2 mg. (women)
Niacin	Dermatitis; insomnia; headache; diarrhea; dementia	18 mg. (men) 13 mg. (women)
Vitamin B_6 (pyridoxine)	Depression; skin lesions; extreme nervousness; water retention; lethargy	2.2 mg. (men) 2.0 mg. (women)
Vitamin B_{12}	Anemia, accompanied by symptoms such as heart palpitations, sore tongue, general weakness; weight loss	3.0 mcg.
Folate	Anemia; dizziness; fatigue; intestinal disorders; diarrhea; shortness of breath	400 mcg.
Vitamin C (ascorbic acid)	Easy bruising; spongy, bleeding gums; dental problems; slow wound healing; fatigue; listlessness; rough skin	60 mg.

Nutrient	Possible Deficiency Symptoms*	RDA for Adults (age 23–50)
Vitamin D	Softening of bones (osteomalacia); bone pain; susceptibility to bone fracture (osteoporosis); excessive tooth decay	200 I.U.
Vitamin E	Muscle degeneration; anemia; nerve dysfunction	15 I.U. (men) 12 I.U. (women)
Calcium	Softening of bones (osteomalacia); susceptibility to bone fracture (osteoporosis); periodontal disease	800 mg.
Iron	Anemia, accompanied by symptoms such as weakness, fatigue, headache, heart palpitations, mouth soreness	10 mg.
Magnesium	Foot and leg cramps; muscle weakness; irregular pulse; nervousness	350 mg. (men) 300 mg. (women)
Zinc	Slow wound healing; skin and hair problems; poor resistance to infection	15 mg.

* These symptoms can, of course, suggest medical conditions other than nutrient deficiencies. For a proper diagnosis of symptoms, see your doctor.

most vitamin and mineral tests sparingly, not routinely. And the consensus in the medical world seems to be that performing nutrient tests on apparently healthy people is a waste of time.

Testing the Tests

And, of course, some nutrient tests can yield more useful data than others.

Calcium tests (done either on blood or urine) are among the most revealing, which may be why they're often included in standard multiple-test batteries. "They're helpful in diagnosing numerous conditions," says Edward R. Pinckney, M.D., a California specialist in preventive medicine and coauthor of *The Patient's Guide to Medical Tests.* "They're used primarily in evaluating suspected abnormalities of the parathyroid gland, memory problems, unusual sleepiness and nerve or muscle dysfunctions. But they can also yield information in the diagnosis of other gland problems (such as lack of adrenal hormones), unexplained bleeding, vitamin D poisoning, osteoporosis, even cancer."

Tests for iron and folate (done on blood only) are especially valuable because they help physicians diagnose anemias, usually those caused by lack of these two nutrients. Iron tests, generally included in multiple-test batteries, are also used to monitor patients on hemodialysis and for tracking down vitamin and other food deficiencies. And folate tests are sometimes used to distinguish between two deficiencies —folate and vitamin B_{12}.

Then there are those nutrient tests of dubious worth. The niacin urine test is one of them, says Dr. Pinckney. "The test is performed to confirm the diagnosis of pellagra, the classic niacin-deficiency disease," he says. "But the symptoms and signs of the disease, plus a successful therapeutic trial of niacin, allow a diagnosis long before the test is needed."

The vitamin B_6 test (done on urine and blood) may have similar problems. "A vitamin B_6 deficiency is usually diagnosed long before a laboratory test confirms it," says Dr. Pinckney. Plus, even when there's no deficiency present, several drugs and diseases can change B_6 levels, rendering the test results suspect.

The Lowdown on Test Results

But regardless of what a test tells you, it's important to remember that test results do not a diagnosis make. They're only a piece of the diagnostic puzzle that your doctor tries to put together. The other pieces are your medical history, health habits, physical exam, age, sex, symptoms, use of medications and more.

It also helps to keep in mind that no medical test is 100 percent reliable. In most medical tests it's always possible, usually in a small percentage of cases, to get "abnormal" test results and still be perfectly healthy or get "normal" results and be sick. "For this reason, you shouldn't worry if your test results do not at first appear to be normal," says endocrinologist Bernard Kliman, M.D., of Massachusetts General Hospital in Boston and coauthor of *What You Should Know about Medical Lab Tests.*

So if you suspect a vitamin or mineral deficiency, should you ask your physician to order nutrient tests? "First of all," Dr. Kliman advises, "don't try to diagnose yourself. That's your doctor's job. Your symptoms could be completely unrelated to a nutrient deficiency or be a deficiency syndrome caused by some secondary disorder. So maybe nutrient tests would be useless—or just what the doctor ordered."

Getting Your Nutrients to Work Better

If you eat three square meals a day or take vitamin supplements, you might think you're getting adequate nutrition. But you could be wrong.

Nutrition isn't that simple or direct. Your body doesn't always make the best use of all the vitamins you take in, either in food or in supplements. Some vitamins never get to where they could do the most good. Others sail through your system without being absorbed.

The same is true of minerals. In fact, when it comes to figuring out how to make the most of your vitamins, minerals are often part of the plan.

If you want to squeeze every available microgram from your vitamins and minerals, it helps to understand some of the ways in which nutrients help each other along.

A Booster Plan for Better Nutrition

Here are some tips to help you make the most of your nutrients.

Eat small, nutritious meals and snacks. All the nutrients your body takes in at a big meal can be hard to swallow, says John Pinto, Ph.D., assistant professor of nutrition and medicine at Cornell University Medical College and associate member at Memorial Sloan-Kettering Cancer Center.

"If you stop and think how some people eat a large amount of protein and carbohydrates at one meal, they really swamp their system with this influx of nutrients all at one time," Dr. Pinto says. "And many of these nutrients won't be absorbed. That's because it's easier for the gastrointestinal tract to absorb nutrients from small amounts of food over a small period of time."

If you want to squeeze more nutritional value from your diet, scale down your main meals and eat healthful snacks—like a piece of fruit, crisp raw vegetables, a whole grain muffin or a glass of milk—in between. You'll give your body a chance to absorb nutrients most efficiently, says Dr. Pinto.

Take your vitamin C in small, divided doses. "The higher your dose at a single time, the smaller the percentage of vitamin C you absorb," explains Mark Levine, M.D., a researcher at the National Institutes of Health in Bethesda, Maryland. "If you take 100 milligrams at one time, you get something like 90 percent absorption. If you go up to a gram [1,000 milligrams], it's approximately 50 percent absorption, and so on."

Instead of taking one large tablet of vitamin C, then, divide the same amount into smaller doses to be taken throughout the day.

"Let's say you chose to take two grams [2,000 milligrams] of vitamin C," says Dr. Levine. "You would increase the percentage of absorption if you took 500 milligrams four times a day or 1,000 milligrams twice a day."

If you want to make sure your iron is more fully absorbed, get more vitamin C. "Vitamin C will enhance absorption of other nutrients, particularly iron," says Dr. Levine.

When we talk about iron, most of us think of foods like beef, poultry, fish and eggs. But not all iron is the same. Only about 10 percent of the iron in vegetables and grain—called nonheme (nonblood) iron—is absorbed. In contrast, we absorb from 15 to 30 percent of the iron found in meats, which is called heme iron.

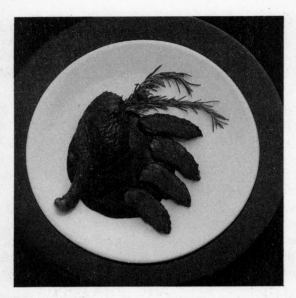

Tomato sauce is more than a tasty complement to meat dishes. Because it contains vitamin C, it can help increase the absorption of iron from your meal.

Vitamin C is what is known as an iron enhancer. It helps convert the nonabsorbed iron into a form the body can use. So to make the most of your iron, eat more foods that are rich in vitamin C, such as tomatoes and oranges, along with iron-rich foods such as lean meat, fish, poultry, leafy green vegetables and whole grains.

One way to improve the absorption of iron in your beef, fish or chicken dish might be to add a thick, spicy tomato sauce. A piece of fruit for dessert, instead of that slab of double-fudge cake you've been coveting, is a healthier alternative if you want to boost your absorption of iron from your meal. If you take an iron supplement, wash it down with a little orange juice.

Special Advice for Vitamins A, D and E

Vitamins A, D and E are absorbed in the intestine in the presence of fat. Consequently, if you take your fat-soluble vitamins on an empty stomach, you might flush out most of the vitamins before they can be absorbed.

Take fat-soluble vitamins with foods that contain fat. "It's reasonable to take fat-soluble vitamins with foods that contain a small amount of fat—for example, a glass of low-fat [1 or 2 percent] milk," says Cedric Garland, Dr.P.H., assistant professor of community and family medicine at the University of California, San Diego. "A moderate amount of fat would cause the secretion of digestive enzymes that work on fats, which would enhance absorption of the fat-soluble vitamins. Without a small amount of fat, a portion of the vitamins will wash right through the intestine without being absorbed."

What about those of us on low-fat diets? Not to worry, says Dr. Garland. "From a practical point of view, a diet containing 15 to 20 percent fat would still be sufficient to absorb fat-soluble vitamins."

Getting the Most Out of Calcium

How and when you get calcium is important.

To move calcium along, get plenty of vitamin D. You can take calcium supplements every day and still leave your bones and teeth crying out for more—if you don't get enough vitamin D along with the mineral. Without vitamin D, calcium is not absorbed.

If you want to make sure you're getting enough of both nutrients, says Dr. Garland, one convenient way to do so is to drink milk, which contains plenty of calcium *and* vitamin D.

But drinking milk is only one way to boost your vitamin D. Perhaps the easiest way for most of us to make sure we get enough vitamin D is to take a stroll in the sunlight. Your skin manufactures vitamin D on its own, but it needs ultraviolet rays from sunlight to start the wheels turning. How much sun do you need to make vitamin D? "Just 15 minutes a day, with sunlight on your hands and face, should be enough in most cases," says Dr. Garland.

The walk will do you good, too, since weight-bearing exercise enhances the movement of calcium to your bones.

Take your calcium with food. Not all of us consume enough dairy products to keep us in calcium balance. If you don't get enough dietary calcium, you might take a supplement, but merely taking a supplement doesn't guarantee you the best results. If you take calcium, it's important to get your gastric juices flowing, because some calcium supplements are absorbed best in an acid environment. (This is also a problem for many people over the age of 60, whose production of stomach acid may be lower.) The solution is to take your calcium with a meal, thus stimulating your stomach to produce enough acid.

Among healthy adults, pregnant and lactating women need the most calcium. The Recommended Dietary Allowance (RDA) for this group is 1,200 milligrams of calcium daily. To get this amount of calcium, you would have to drink four or five glasses of milk a day. People who are at risk for osteoporosis may need even more, although the precise amount hasn't been firmly established.

Food also helps improve the absorption of other nutrients. "It's best that nutrients be consumed with a meal," says Dr. Pinto. "The very sight of food begins to stimulate the appetite, triggering the release of various enzymes. Also, hormonal responses begin to register. With food in the mouth, insulin rises. Intestinal blood flow increases, preparing to help transport food through the body and move nutrients from the intestine into the bloodstream."

Take your calcium supplements before bed.   The timing of the dose could improve your body's absorption of the mineral, too. Morris Notelovitz, M.D., medical director of the Climacteric Clinic in Gainesville, Florida, has suggested taking calcium supplements just before you turn in.

During the day, your body extracts the calcium it needs from food. At night, when no food is coming in, your body still needs to maintain normal blood levels of calcium, so it raids the only source available to it—your skeleton.

A calcium supplement just before bed should keep your blood levels near normal and protect your bones from this nightly pilferage. But if you're going to take calcium, remember the previous advice and swallow it with a glass of low-fat milk to stimulate the production of stomach acids.

New Discoveries in Mineral Nutrition

Time was, folks used to drink water warmed up with a red-hot sword as a means of getting their daily iron. That was well before people fully understood what iron was or why they needed it. It probably didn't taste very good, but early medicine men obviously were on the cutting edge of mineral nutrition. They were able to figure out that the metal from that saber somehow perked people up.

Even so, it has taken medical science literally centuries to probe the health benefits of minerals. Over the last hundred years or so, researchers have started to catch up.

Most of us know a little bit about certain minerals. We've lived through a lifetime of television ads warning about the perils of "iron-poor blood." Lately we've been hearing and reading about calcium deficiency and osteoporosis, the brittle-bones disease that afflicts women and the elderly.

But what of selenium, copper, potassium and chromium? Are these really nutrients or are they what you have left over when you melt down a '65 Ford Falcon?

Research scientists continue to unearth new and intriguing information about these and many other "rare earths." Here are some of the most recent developments.

Magnesium

Your bones, nerves and teeth need magnesium. So do your muscles, especially your heart muscle. Magnesium plays a part in keeping it beating rhythmically.

But much of the Western world doesn't get enough magnesium, and the result could be a higher incidence of heart disease and hypertension. That's because many areas are served by a soft-water drinking supply, which lacks the magnesium content of hard water.

People living in hard-water areas may bemoan the fact that their soap won't lather readily. On the other hand, the incidence of heart-disease-related death is 10.1 percent lower there than in soft-water regions, according to the journal *Magnesium.*

Additionally, studies show a relationship between low magnesium levels and high blood pressure and stroke.

Magnesium deficiency may adversely affect your ability to stand up to long periods of vigorous exercise. At the University of California at Davis, rats fed a magnesium-deficient diet ran out of gas faster than their brother rats, who consumed a normal diet—normal for rodents, that is. This research suggests that the rats' exercise capacity declined along with the magnesium in their diet.

It is far too soon to tell what impact this new research will have on humans. But studies are under way at Davis to explore the effects of magnesium deficiency on people. This continuing research could provide some insight into the impact of magnesium deficiency on the human immune system as well.

People who attempt suicide may have low levels of magnesium in the cerebrospinal fluid, according to research from the Regional Neuropsychiatric Institute in Hungary. Magnesium is thought to be necessary for the release of serotonin, a neurotransmitter that strikes a balance between manic and depressed behavior.

In several studies, magnesium has been reported useful in controlling premature labor and fetal growth retardation. This doesn't apply to all expectant mothers but to those at particular risk for premature delivery. It has been theorized that magnesium deficiency disturbs the delicate metabolism of the placenta.

Patients who receive radiation therapy for cervical cancer sometimes find that the treatment involves damage to the colon, leading to chronic diarrhea. Israeli researchers found that intravenous magnesium, along with antidiarrhea drugs, alleviated the diarrhea. They theorize that radiation decreases serum magnesium levels. In turn, diarrhea may be a result of magnesium deficiency.

Previous research has laid the groundwork for these provocative new theories.

"There's a lot more to this than just subjective ideas," according to Burton M. Altura, Ph.D., professor of physiology at Downstate Medical Center in Brooklyn and founder of the American Society for Magnesium Research. "Now we have a lot of objectivity, a lot of good scientific work being done. This isn't to say that all these things will pass the test of time. But certainly, the cardiovascular aspects that have come to the forefront over the last five to seven years are valid and are going to be extremely useful in the diagnosis and treatment of patients with various types of cardiovascular ailments." Full-blown magnesium deficiency is not common in the West, says Dr. Altura. The problem, he says, is borderline deficiency.

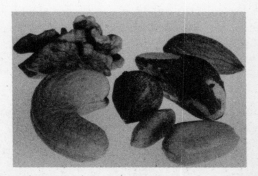

Nuts provide a bounty of minerals — magnesium, copper, calcium and zinc — that are essential for many important body functions.

"It's a serious problem," he adds. "The public must become aware of this and must attempt to have a balanced diet."

The Recommended Dietary Allowance (RDA) for magnesium is from 300 milligrams for women to 350 milligrams for men. Nuts and whole grain cereals are good food sources of magnesium.

Copper

Some women who suffer frequent miscarriages early in pregnancy are low in copper. Recent research suggests a strong connection.

"This was a very serendipitous observation," says Maryann Breskin, a research associate in the Department of Nutrition at the University of Washington. "We were looking at something else—zinc and copper levels throughout pregnancy. We realized that some of these girls who were losing their babies sometimes had low copper levels."

Previous animal studies have established the relationship between zinc and copper and fetal malformation, Breskin says.

Copper helps your body absorb iron. Copper deficiency can lead to skeletal malformation and albinism. Also, the rare genetic Menke's disease, known as "kinky hair syndrome," results from genetic inability to absorb copper. The mineral plays a part in fertility and in the formation of hemoglobin. Copper deficiency also has been linked to high serum cholesterol levels.

The National Academy of Sciences, which sets the RDAs, recommends from two to three milligrams of copper daily for adults and roughly half that amount for children. Nuts, seeds, red meats, liver and organ meats are good sources of this mineral.

Selenium

Selenium, along with vitamin E, significantly improved the outlook of 15 elderly patients in a rest home in Finland. According to researchers, after a year of vitamin E and selenium, the patients were more alert, less anxious or hostile and better able to care for themselves.

Selenium also is an antioxidant, a cancer fighter and immune system stimulator. The National Academy of Sciences suggests a daily intake of 50 to 200 micrograms for adults. Fish, whole grains and organ meats are excellent sources of selenium.

Calcium

Calcium helps build up your bones and helps prevent osteoporosis. Postmenopausal women, in particular, may lose 2 to 4 percent of their bone mass per year during the first eight to ten years after menopause. Even a 1 percent loss can lead to higher risks for broken bones, researchers say.

Exercise helps speed the calcium along on its way to your skeleton. When you're inactive, your body decides you don't need as much calcium, and the mineral is flushed out of your bones, a little at a time.

Of all the minerals in your body, calcium is king. There's more of it than of any other mineral. Without it, your blood wouldn't clot, your teeth would turn to mush and your heart would beat to a different drummer.

We also know that men consume more calcium-bearing foods than women do. It's thought to be one reason women are more at risk for osteoporosis.

The adult RDA for calcium is 800 milligrams in adults. Cheese is a rich source. So are other dairy products, nuts, green vegetables and sardines.

Potassium

Researchers at the University of Minnesota Hospital and Medical School found that lab rats with high blood pressure had fewer fatal strokes when potassium was added to their diet. This was true even though blood pressure remained about the same.

That's fine for hypertensive rats, but what about people? This study suggests that increased potassium in the human diet could reduce the occurrence of potentially fatal brain hemorrhages.

Potassium also keeps your ticker in sync. Your pancreas needs potassium, too, in order to secrete insulin.

Fresh fruits and vegetables—bananas, tomatoes, celery, cabbage and grapefruit, to name a few—are excellent sources of potassium.

Zinc

High levels of stress may lead to temporary zinc deficiency. In one study, hospital patients awaiting surgery showed clinical signs of deficiency in the form of dermatitis. The rashes, scaly skin and ulcers responded well to oral zinc supplements and zinc oxide ointment.

Zinc sulfate solutions may prevent oral and genital herpes. William W. Halcomb, D.O., of Austin, Texas, has reviewed research on zinc and herpes. He says the antiherpes claims appear to be accurate, although there still is no definitive cure. "Zinc either prevents or slows down multiplication of the herpes virus, for reasons not clearly understood," says Dr. Halcomb. "The lesions heal in a shorter time."

Zinc, it seems, truly is the nutrient of many faces, playing a role in the maintenance of male fertility, disease resistance, brain development and cell growth. It helps your gums resist the harmful effects of dental plaque. Without zinc in your diet, even your taste buds take a snooze. Food doesn't taste good.

If you have a wound or burn, zinc helps it heal. Your skin needs zinc, too. If you see white spots on your fingernails, it could be a sign you aren't getting enough zinc. The RDA for zinc is 15 milligrams daily. Food sources include liver and beef. Popcorn, cheddar cheese and peanuts are good sources, too.

Does Your Multiple Add Up?

Have you ever stared at a store shelf full of vitamin bottles, totally bewildered? With visions of brightly colored pills spinning through your head, you might well wish for an easier way. Could a multiple vitamin/mineral formula be just the thing you need?

A multiple combines many nutrients into one tablet or capsule. It's for people who don't want to take several different vitamin pills each day. Then, if it falls short here or there (you may have some special needs), it's easy enough to supplement with additional individual nutrients.

Choosing the multivitamin that's best for you requires a bit of comparison shopping. You need to know how vitamin and mineral supplements meet, or miss, your particular nutrient needs. Here's a step-by-step guide.

Start with the Essentials

One of the best things you can do is compare the list of nutrients on a vitamin bottle label with the U.S. Recommended Daily Allowances (USRDAs). Take the table on page 28, What to Look For in a Multivitamin, with you to the store. Compare the label with the table, item for item. Does the multiple include all of the vitamins and minerals listed in the table? It should. These are the basic ingredients of good nutrition.

Some essential nutrients, especially trace elements, do not yet have USRDAs. They do have safe and accepted ranges, which are also listed in the table.

How many of these nutrients are in the multiple? You may not feel you need every one, but you should know which you want, and why. You may want chromium if you're concerned about diabetes, since chromium seems to play a role in glucose metabolism; selenium, a potent antioxidant, because of its possible role in cancer protection; copper if you're taking supplemental zinc. (Copper is important in the formation of red blood cells and capillary stability. Zinc may affect copper absorption. Look for a ratio of about 7.5 to 10 units of zinc to 1 portion of copper. For example, 15 milligrams of zinc should be taken with 2 milligrams of copper.)

You may find many other ingredients—from bioflavonoids to tin—in multiple vitamins. While it's true that these substances are found naturally in food, research has not determined any of them to be essential to human nutrition, at least not yet.

Decide How Much You Need

You also should look at the amount of each nutrient in the supplement, measured in milligrams, micrograms (1/1000 of a milligram) or international units. Compare each with the USRDA amounts. In addition to amounts, most labels list a nutrient's percentages of the USRDA, and this may actually provide you with the best information regarding the product's potency and balance, as you'll see below.

How potent a multiple do you want? If your goal is "insurance," look for those providing 50 to 150 percent of the USRDA. The American Medical Association generally considers this a reasonable range, with one important exception: The vitamin D level should not exceed 100 percent.

Some, but certainly not all, "one-tablet-daily" types are in this category. If you want more than the USRDA, "high-potency" brands may provide it. But so will some other multiples without these labels, says Sheldon Hendler, M.D., Ph.D., formerly clinical instructor of medicine at the University of California at San Diego, author of *The Complete Guide to Anti-Aging Nutrients.*

Check Nutritional Balance

Look at the percentage of the USRDA of each nutrient. If the formula is balanced by USRDA standards, each nutrient will have the same percentage of the USRDA. A balanced multiple may contain 100 percent of the USRDA for each nutrient, for instance. If it's not balanced, some percentages will be high, some low. That's not necessarily bad. But you should note how it varies and decide if that's something you want.

Some "women's formulas," for instance, contain additional iron or calcium to accommodate increased needs for those nutrients among many women. Some "geri," or geriatric, formulas have additional antioxidants—vitamins A, E and C and selenium—nutrients believed to play a role in slowing some aspects of aging.

Most of the so-called stress formulas provide much more vitamin C and B complex, and sometimes zinc, than they do other nutrients (because of their purported role in beating stress). Other formulas, like B-100 types, provide nutrients in increments of 100 milligrams or 100 micrograms. As a result, the formulas may be far out of balance, since the USRDAs for some B vitamins are less than one-tenth that of other B vitamins.

"I personally think these products play on the fact that people don't know what 'balanced' is," says Annette Dickinson, technical counselor of the Council for Responsible Nutrition, a vitamin manufacturers' trade association. "It makes no sense to have some of the B vitamins present at 100 times the USRDA, others at only a fraction of the USRDA."

Beware of Advertising Claims

There are now supplement formulas for almost every medical condition you can imagine—arthritis, high blood pressure, heart disease, depression, fatigue, premenstrual discomfort and so forth.

"Be extremely wary of any formula that claims to counteract any particular disease," Dr. Hendler says. "Most of the special formulas I've surveyed are very poorly designed. I think you're better off sticking with a good basic regimen."

But, with your doctor's advice, you may want to take additional vitamins or minerals for a medical problem. If you're a woman, you may take additional iron for anemia or additional calcium to prevent osteoporosis.

If you have a leg-cramping condition called intermittent claudication, your doctor might suggest extra vitamin E. Or he may prescribe extra B_6 and magnesium to help prevent kidney stones or larger-than-normal amounts of vitamin C for bronchial asthma. In this sense, the vitamins are going beyond the role of nutrition. They are acting almost as drugs, in a therapeutic sense. Their advantage is that they often have fewer side effects than drugs used for these same conditions. But they still need to be used wisely and under a doctor's supervision. And typically, multiples are not the best way because the target nutrient is mixed with many others.

Does Your Multiple Have a Deficiency?

Some vitamin manufacturers add inadequate amounts of nutrients to their products just so they can list the nutrient on their label, Dr. Hendler says. And even the better products sometimes contain only small amounts of some nutrients. Here again, it's important to read the label.

The once-daily multiple vitamin/mineral supplements are often low in calcium and magnesium because these two nutrients are bulky and make the pill big. There are many individual calcium supplements on the market to make up the difference, though. You can also find some good calcium/magnesium products, which provide what some researchers think is an important 2.5 to 1 ratio of these two minerals. (Magnesium is an important mineral for calcium metabolism.) If you are taking calcium to prevent or treat osteoporosis, you should know that some researchers think trace minerals, such as zinc and copper, are very important for bones, too.

Other Shopping Tips

Here are some other things to be aware of as you choose a supplement.

Check the expiration date. Many, but not all, vitamin manufacturers now include an expiration date on their products. It's a good idea to avoid a product beyond the expiration date, although most products retain their potency much longer. Oil-based supplements deteriorate more quickly than others. If you're selecting products from a store's discount bin, check to see that the vitamins aren't leftovers from the Stone Age.

Too much to swallow? Some manufacturers who try to cram everything into a once-daily tablet do so at the expense of your esophagus. Check the pill size before you buy. Sometimes the better choice is to get a just-as-complete but smaller multiple that must be taken not once but two or three times a day.

More is not better. You may be tempted to think that if your multiple at its suggested dosage isn't good enough, you can just take it more often and not bother to switch to some better-balanced product. You may want more calcium, for instance, but you would need to take three pills daily, rather than one, to get it from your present supplement. "Don't do that," Dr. Hendler emphasizes. "Taking an unbalanced supplement three times a day still may not provide the recommended doses of some nutrients, but you may end up taking too much of other nutrients, throwing things even farther out of balance."

Do your homework. You can do some comparison shopping before you go to the store by looking through the *Handbook of Nonprescription Drugs,* published by the American Pharmaceutical Association, Washington, DC 20037 (found in the reference section of large libraries, especially those affiliated with medical schools). This book contains a table of many multiple vitamin products, their ingredients and amounts. The table is a good way to do some comparison shopping for supplements before you head for the store.

What to Look For in a Multivitamin

Nutrient	USRDA (adults and children 4 or more years of age)
Vitamin A	5,000 I.U.
Thiamine (B_1)	1.5 mg.
Riboflavin (B_2)	1.7 mg.
Niacin	20 mg.
Vitamin B_6 (pyridoxine)	2 mg.
Vitamin B_{12}	6 mcg.
Folate	0.4 mg.
Biotin	300 mcg.
Pantothenate	10 mg.
Vitamin C (ascorbic acid)	60 mg.
Vitamin D	400 I.U.
Vitamin E	30 I.U.
Calcium	1,000 mg.
Copper	2 mg.
Iodine	150 mcg.
Iron	18 mg.
Magnesium	400 mg.
Phosphorus	1,000 mg.
Zinc	15 mg.
	Suggested Ranges*
Chromium	50-200 mcg.
Selenium	50-200 mcg.[†]

*These nutrients are considered essential, but they have no USRDA. Instead, they have ranges that are considered safe and adequate.

[†]Supplements of selenium should not exceed 100 mcg., since the average diet supplies about 100 mcg.

B Alert

Aunt Mary wasn't all that old when her husband died—only 65—but in the past three years it seems as though she's aged 20 years, at least as far as her mind goes. She's forgetful, irritable and tired. And some days she's so confused, it's heartbreaking. You hate to think she's becoming senile, but what else could it be?

Teenagers are supposed to be rebellious, it's true, but you're beginning to wonder if your 14-year-old daughter's moodiness and hyperactivity aren't above and beyond normal adolescent turmoil. You're also wondering how anyone can live on french fries and soft drinks, which are about the only foods she'll eat these days. Could that be part of the problem?

The divorce was hard on Tim, but he was determined to pick up and go on with his life. Instead, though, he began feeling so emotionally and physically exhausted he found it hard to do his job, much less look after himself. Instead of getting better, Tim is slowly getting worse. Could the stress be catching up with him?

Nutrition-oriented doctors see these kinds of cases again and again, in different combinations of the same factors—aging, long-term stress, poor eating habits, even special metabolic needs. They also see the unfortunate consequences. Aunt Mary could end up in a nursing home before her time, that wall-climbing teenager might become a high-school dropout, and perhaps Tim will find himself severely depressed, even suicidal.

But all three share a common problem—a B-complex vitamin deficiency. And they all could have gotten relief from their mental woes—perhaps prevented them altogether—if they'd been getting enough of these nutrients to meet their personal needs.

When Stress Runs High, B Vitamins Run Low

"Take someone who's just a little depressed or a little stressed because of things going on in his life. That person might find himself eating poorly. And that could lead to nutritional deficiencies that push him over the brink, into true depression or mental problems," says Charles Tkacz, M.D., medical director of the North Nassau Mental Health Center in Manhasset, New York. The center's specialty is finding and correcting nutritional deficiencies in psychiatric patients, an aspect of treatment that's all too often overlooked in traditional medical care.

Robert Picker, M.D., a Walnut Creek, California, psychiatrist, agrees. "I've run into this kind of situation too many times to count," he says. "The body's nutritional needs are increased during times of stress. What may normally be adequate suddenly becomes a deficiency. And that deficiency could begin a vicious circle of mental symptoms that the person just doesn't seem to be able to shake. In fact, as a psychiatrist, I am painfully aware that many of these people are in psychotherapy for long periods of time without ever realizing that the correction of a nutritional deficiency could have significantly helped or possibly cured their problem, or perhaps have prevented it in the first place."

Overall nutrition is essential, but doctors should take a special look at the B-complex vitamins, especially B_6, B_{12}, thiamine (vitamin B_1), niacin and folate.

Why are the B vitamins important for our mental health? The brain, it seems, is more sensitive to fluctuations in dietary nutrients than neurologists once thought. It has a special need for B vitamins to perform at its best.

The role of B vitamins is extensive and complex. They are co-enzymes, or catalysts, in many of the body's most basic functions, including the process of oxidation, or the body's burning of food to provide fuel. What this means is that they're needed to supply the brain with its energy source—glucose. Without enough glucose, the brain begins to perform poorly. Fatigue, depression, even hallucinations can be symptoms of a low glucose level in the brain. B_6 and niacin are the B vitamins most involved in this process.

Low Levels of B Vitamins Can Lead to Confusion

But the B vitamins play a second crucial role in our mental health. Several are known to be involved in the production of neurotransmitters, biochemicals that allow the brain cells to pass messages along their nerve pathways.

"B_6 is needed for the production of serotonin, a major neurotransmitter in many body functions," says Eric Braverman, M.D., of the Princeton Brain Bio Center in Skillman, New Jersey. "Folate helps produce catecholamines, which control many body functions. B_{12} is needed to produce acetylcholine, another neurotransmitter. In other words, all the chemicals produced by the brain cells depend on nutrients taken into the body, and in many cases, they seem to depend on certain B vitamins."

What happens when they're not there?

"We know that people who aren't getting enough of these nutrients get a whole host of psychiatric and neurological symptoms, like depression, confusion, fatigue and psychosis," Dr. Tkacz says.

It was seeing that volunteers deprived of B_6 soon sank into a funk, that prisoners of war fed thiamine-poor polished rice lost muscle coordination and reasoning power, and that diets short on B_{12} or folate could cause symptoms of senility or psychosis that led doctors to begin thinking backward. If nutrient deficiencies caused such problems, perhaps people with these symptoms could be helped with doses of the nutrients they seemed to be missing.

That's exactly what doctors like Dr. Tkacz, Dr. Braverman and

Dr. Picker are doing. "We take blood samples for special nutritional testing, then initially put most patients on therapeutic doses of many nutrients, including 40 to 50 milligrams a day of all the B vitamins," Dr. Tkacz says. When the nutritional tests have been evaluated, the patient may be given more of a specific vitamin, mineral or amino acid that's been found to be lacking in his body.

"We've found, and studies confirm, that many depressed patients

Depressed People May Have a B_6 Deficiency

Seriously depressed patients may have another problem to contend with, according to Jonathan W. Stewart, M.D., of the New York State Psychiatric Institute and Columbia University College of Physicians and Surgeons. "About 20 percent of the depressed patients we looked at showed neurological symptoms as well—numbness and tingling in the hands, like 'pins and needles' or 'electric shock' sensations. And those with the symptoms had significantly lower vitamin B_6 levels than did those without symptoms.

"I feel quite certain that low vitamin B_6 levels are responsible for these neurological symptoms," Dr. Stewart says. "What we don't know yet is whether the low vitamin B_6 levels are in fact causing the depression. It's conceivable that B_6 has a role because the enzyme processes that convert foodstuffs into neurotransmitters [chemicals in the body that carry electrical signals from nerve to nerve] require vitamin B_6 at several critical stages. In B_6 deficiency, patients might not produce enough neurotransmitters, which in turn could lead to the symptoms of depression."

If a patient is admitted with both depression and neurological symptoms, the possibility of B_6 deficiency should be considered, says Dr. Stewart. "B_6 may relieve the neurological symptoms, and we suspect it may even have a positive effect on depression."

are low in B_6," Dr. Tkacz says. "A certain number are helped to recover from their depression by taking B_6 under medical supervision."

Bad Nerves? Check for Thiamine

Derrick Lonsdale, M.D., a Cleveland physician with a special interest in biochemistry and nutrition, found that one of the first signs of a thiamine deficiency was changes in behavior—neurotic symptoms like depression, insomnia, chest pain and chronic fatigue. All 20 of the patients he studied improved with additional thiamine.

Not incidentally, these nervous patients also had poor diets. They were eating lots of "empty calories," usually refined carbohydrates or sugar-laden drinks, foods that used up their thiamine reserves without putting any back, Dr. Lonsdale reports.

Folate Deficiency and Depression

And several doctors are looking into folate deficiency as a cause of depression, insomnia, irritability, forgetfulness and some supposedly psychosomatic disorders.

In reviewing medical literature, A. Missagh Ghadirian, M.D., of the Royal Victoria Hospital, Montreal, found folate-deficiency depression in people taking antibiotics, birth control pills, anticonvulsants and medications for rheumatoid arthritis. "Sometimes the deficiencies are quite severe, but sometimes they are more marginal and might even escape notice," he says. "If the depression is due to deficiency, making sure the patient gets enough additional folate works well to relieve the condition."

Mental Woes Linked to Low B_{12}

Doctors are realizing now, too, that sometimes the first sign of a B_{12} deficiency can be bizarre mental misfirings that resemble psychosis or senility. One 47-year-old woman who had been "seeing" flying saucers was found to have low B_{12} levels. Four days after starting B_{12} supplementation, her hallucinations were gone.

One of Dr. Tkacz's patients was a confused, forgetful woman in her early sixties. She'd been diagnosed as senile, but her family had decided to check for a nutritional deficiency. It turned out the woman

Low on B Vitamins?

How many of these risk factors for a B vitamin deficiency fit you?

- You eat a diet that's high in sugar.
- You seldom eat liver, brewer's yeast or whole grains.
- You've been under a lot of stress lately.
- You have digestion problems or have had stomach or small intestine surgery.
- You take any one of these: birth control pills, diuretics, cholesterol-lowering drugs, antibiotics, psychoactive or anticonvulsant drugs.
- You drink alcohol regularly.
- You drink a lot of coffee.
- You smoke cigarettes.

Do you have any of these symptoms?

- You feel more tired, irritable, depressed, emotional, irrational or anxious than you'd like or than you think is normal.
- You are older and have suddenly developed emotional or mental problems, especially depression, even though you have no prior history of any mental problems.
- Counseling and psychotherapy haven't helped your problems.
- You have skin rashes that won't go away.
- You have sores inside your mouth or cracks around the corners of your mouth.
- You have numbness, tingling or twitching in your legs, or your feet burn.
- You suffer from premenstrual tension or postpartum depression.

Note: These problems may well have causes other than, or besides, B-vitamin deficiency. Work out the solution with a good physician.

had a very low level of B_{12}, and with just a few injections she recovered completely, Dr. Tkacz says. "She'll have to have B_{12} injections for the rest of her life, but that's certainly better than being prematurely consigned to a nursing home.

"A lot of families would have simply written off her symptoms as part of aging, but that's not usually the case," Dr. Tkacz adds. "That's why it's so important to be careful when you're dealing with a possible diagnosis of dementia or Alzheimer's disease. You want to make sure you're not dealing with a B_{12} or a folate deficiency. I'd say 5 to 10 percent, easily, of elderly people with mental problems really have nutritional deficiencies, and many involve the B-complex vitamins."

Beware the "Tea and Toast" Syndrome

It's the borderline B-vitamin deficiencies that are most likely to slip through the cracks of traditional medicine—those that might present themselves only as depression, fatigue and irritability, which are symptoms for which most doctors would find no cause.

"I think the borderline deficiencies are extremely common," Dr. Tkacz says. "It's what's called the 'tea and toast' syndrome. Older people living on Social Security or a pension find themselves short of money and don't eat as well as they should." Add to that teenagers subsisting on fast foods and people of any age who let life's stresses overtake their daily intake of B vitamins, and you've got quite a crowd.

So what's the best protection? Eating foods rich in the B-complex vitamins is important. (See the table, Best Food Sources of B Vitamins, on pages 36 and 37 for a list of good sources.) Whole grains, peanuts, seeds and beans also contain good amounts. An alternative is B_{12}-fortified brewer's yeast or a good B-complex supplement.

"I have my patients take from one teaspoon to one tablespoon of brewer's yeast a day," Dr. Picker says. He also has them follow a diet that's high in fiber and complex carbohydrates and low in fats and sweets. "I advise them to minimize or eliminate alcohol or caffeine intake, and I always give them a big lecture about smoking. All three of those are big users of the B vitamins."

"Just one simple step of providing B complex or brewer's yeast in the diet can eliminate a whole host of potential neurological and psychological problems," adds Dr. Tkacz.

Best Food Sources of B Vitamins

Food	Portion	Thiamine (mg.)	Riboflavin (mg.)	Niacin (mg.)	B₆ (mg.)	B₁₂ (mcg.)	Folate (mcg.)
Beef, round, full cut, separable lean only, cooked	3 oz.	0.086	0.195	3.540	0.430	2.53	9
Beef kidneys, simmered	3 oz.	0.162	3.450	5.110	0.440	43.60	83
Beef liver, braised	3 oz.	0.167	3.480	9.110	0.770	60.35	185
Brewer's yeast	1 tbsp.	1.250	0.340	3.000	0.200	0.00	313
Brown rice, raw	¼ cup	0.170	0.030	2.350	0.280	0.00	8
Chicken, light meat, cooked	3 oz.	0.060	0.100	10.560	0.510	0.29	3
Chicken liver, cooked	3 oz.	0.130	1.490	3.780	0.500	16.49	654
Chick-peas, boiled	½ cup	0.095	0.052	0.431	0.114	0.00	141
Egg, hard-cooked	1	0.040	0.140	0.030	0.060	0.66	24
Kidney beans, all types, boiled	½ cup	0.141	0.051	0.509	0.106	0.00	114
Milk, whole	1 cup	0.090	0.400	0.210	0.100	0.87	12

Navy beans, boiled	½ cup	0.184	0.056	0.483	0.149	0.00	127
Peanuts, all types, dry-roasted	¼ cup	0.000	0.035	4.930	0.093	0.00	53
Rye flour	¼ cup	0.200	0.070	0.880	0.100	0.00	17
Salmon steak, cooked	3 oz.	0.150	0.060	8.400	0.640	2.95	18
Soybeans, boiled	½ cup	0.133	0.245	0.343	0.201	0.00	46
Sunflower seeds, dry	¼ cup	0.820	0.090	1.620	0.450	0.00	85
Swiss cheese	2 oz.	0.010	0.210	0.050	0.050	0.95	4
Wheat germ, toasted	1 tbsp.	0.120	0.060	0.400	0.070	0.00	25
Whole wheat flour	¼ cup	0.170	0.040	1.300	0.100	0.00	16

SOURCES: Adapted from

Agriculture Handbook Nos. 8-1, 8-5, 8-8, 8-12, 8-13, 8-16, 456 (Washington. D.C.: U.S. Department of Agriculture).

"Folacin in Selected Foods," by Betty P. Perloff and R. R. Butrum, *Journal of American Dietetic Association*, February 1977.

Pantothenic Acid, Vitamin B_6 and Vitamin B_{12}, Home Economics Research Report No. 36. by Martha Louise Orr (Washington. D.C.: Agricultural Research Service. U.S. Department of Agriculture. 1969).

A Vitamin C Update

Consider these reports from the medical news grapevine:

- Eighty women seeking Pap smears at the Bronx Municipal Hospital Center may have helped medical science narrow down one of the causes of cervical cancer.
- At a medical research institution in Philadelphia, a laboratory experiment turned up unexpected results that may someday lead to much-needed relief for rheumatoid arthritis sufferers.
- A leading cancer journal has reported evidence supporting the role of a key food element in relief of certain kinds of cancer.
- From 1964 to 1978, consumption of vegetables and fruits high in a particular nutrient increased. At the same time, cardiovascular deaths declined. And at least one medical researcher thinks it was no coincidence.

The surprising common denominator, in all cases, is vitamin C. Although you may have considered vitamin C, or ascorbic acid, essential to everyday good health, a growing body of medical evidence suggests this versatile nutrient may play a more important role in the prevention of disease. Much of this new information is still in the theoretical stage, but it is intriguing. Here's a wrap-up of recent developments. (See the table on page 45 for some sources of vitamin C in the diet.)

Vitamin C May Keep Cervical Dysplasia in Check

A low dietary intake of vitamin C is related to cervical abnormalities. That's what Seymour Romney, M.D., found when he tallied up the results of tests comparing women with normal Pap smears and those with cervical cancer or dysplasia—abnormal cell growth that may or may not lead to cancer.

Of the 80 women at the Bronx Municipal Hospital Center who had Pap smears taken, 34 had normal results. Their dietary intake of vitamin C was relatively high. The remaining 46 women took in considerably less vitamin C in the diet, and their diagnoses ranged from mild cervical inflammation to cancer.

Just a coincidence—or a connection? While there's still a lot of work to be done, Dr. Romney believes there is a definite relationship between cervical cancer and low vitamin C in the diet.

"A lot of people have been intrigued by the prospect that vitamin C may have antitumor properties, and there are reasonable scientific studies that support that idea," explains Dr. Romney.

How and why vitamin C may prevent tumors from forming isn't well understood, however. In fact, says Dr. Romney, vitamin C is probably just one part of the picture.

"Cancer is a terribly complicated disease," he says. "With regard to the role of any nutrients, their actions surely involve interactions with other chemicals in the body, which need to be looked into. It's not likely that a single nutrient, per se, is the cause and effect of a disease as complex as cancer."

The preliminary research suggests that women may not be getting enough vitamin C to prevent cervical cancer. Why? Because, says Dr. Romney, "If there's a disorder in the cervix, that increases the demand for ascorbic acid."

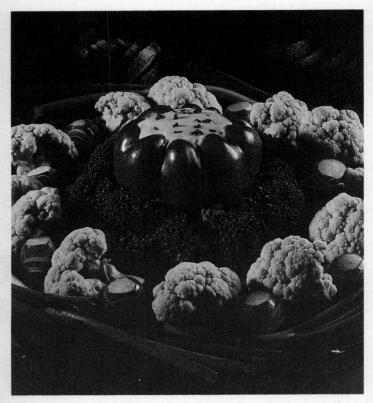

Broccoli and cauliflower are only two of the many good food sources of vitamin C. The fact that this vitamin may be able to prevent certain types of cancer, relieve arthritis and reduce the risk of heart disease makes it a nutrient that no one should be without.

Whether you need more than the Recommended Dietary Allowance (RDA) of 60 milligrams of vitamin C daily just isn't clear. However, Dr. Romney and his research staff would like to find out. "We're going to try to get some solid information on dosage and the effects of that dosage, whether there are side effects and how well it works."

Vitamin C versus Nitrosamines

Of course, cervical cancer is just one of many cancers, and research continues to determine how vitamin C affects other types of cancer, too.

You might have heard about the link between vitamin C and nitrosamines, cancer-causing substances formed by the interaction of nitrite—a common food additive—and chemicals in your body.

Vitamin C has long been believed to prevent nitrosamines from forming. A study reported in the journal *Carcinogenesis* lends strong support to that theory.

Researchers in Britain asked eight volunteers to take a gram (1,000 milligrams) of vitamin C every day for a week. Before and after the experiment, researchers siphoned off gastric juice from the volunteers' stomachs. In all but one of the volunteers, levels of nitrosamines in the gastric juice were significantly lower at the end of the test.

Does this mean vitamin C prevents gastric cancer? No, but it may reduce the risk. Are the results definitive—that is, is this the last word? No. Further studies, and on a wider scale, should be done before coming to any definite conclusions. But the results of this study do give reason for optimism.

Relief for Arthritis— without Side Effects

Picture the body at war with itself. That's what happens in rheumatoid arthritis. The body's own cells mistake body tissues for foreign substances. To repel the "invaders," the cells manufacture antibodies to attack the tissue.

There is no cure for rheumatoid arthritis. Treatment often involves using steroids to reduce the pain and tissue swelling brought about by this disfiguring disease. But these anti-inflammatory drugs in themselves can cause side effects.

That's why Robert H. Davis, Ph.D., a professor in the Department of Physiology at the Pennsylvania College of Podiatric Medicine, has been exploring the use of vitamin C and aloe, two natural substances that cause few if any known side effects.

"It's an idea that goes back, for me, almost 30 years," says Dr. Davis. "Steroids and synthetic drugs have their place in the treatment of arthritis, but the side effects can sometimes be worse than the cure."

Why vitamin C? Simply because, says Dr. Davis, vitamin C is an essential building block in the manufacture of the connective tissue called collagen. In rheumatoid arthritis, this connective tissue breaks down. But Dr. Davis believes that vitamin C, applied to the skin, may prevent or slow this tissue breakdown, reducing inflammation. And aloe also is believed to have healing properties.

In a prize-winning study that put his theory to the test, Dr. Davis and two students combined vitamin C, aloe and ribonucleic acid—a cellular building block also thought to reduce inflammation—in a

A Little Vitamin C May Go a Long Way

Elderly people with low vitamin C levels in their blood are usually given heavy doses of the vitamin to bring their plasma levels up to normal. Now a group of researchers in England says that may be overkill. A little vitamin C may go a long way.

Researchers at the University of Leeds and High Royds Hospital found that low blood levels usually meant low intake of foods rich in vitamin C—in part because of food preparation procedures in institutions and dental problems that made eating fruit impossible for the older people.

But by simply adding fresh orange juice or a vitamin C tablet to the diet—no more than the Recommended Dietary Allowance of 60 milligrams a day—the scientists found they could bring those elderly people who had marginal deficiencies up to normal. Those with deficiencies in the scurvy range, the researchers said, obviously need a larger dose. However, they added, evidence indicates there are far more elderly at risk of marginal deficiencies, which have their own potential health consequences, such as delayed healing of injuries.

cream ointment. Then they applied the cream to the arthritic hind paws of laboratory rats. The results were surprising. Joint-tissue swelling was reduced dramatically, both in the early stages of arthritis and later on, after the disease had progressed for several days. "I honestly didn't think it would work," says Dr. Davis. "But I was able to repeat the results."

Of course, it is too soon to say what impact these studies will have on humans. Furthermore, it's important to understand that this report doesn't suggest that vitamin C is a cure for rheumatoid arthritis. But it offers some hope for an effective treatment that doesn't rely on steroids.

"I wouldn't recommend this kind of treatment to anyone until we get some real statistical data," says Dr. Davis. "I would like to say yes because rheumatoid arthritis is one of the tough ones. But I think it first has to go into a clinical trial and be evaluated. If somebody has a real bad case of arthritis, they should be treated by a doctor."

Vitamin C Up, Heart Disease Down

Most animals make their own vitamin C. In fact, there are only a few species—humans, guinea pigs, monkeys and certain fruit bats —that have to get their vitamin C from what they eat.

Members of the one civilized, self-aware species in that group appear to suffer a chronic dietary shortage of vitamin C, says Anthony Verlangieri, Ph.D., of the University of Mississippi. "And because of that deficiency," he says, "they may be more susceptible to heart disease."

Dr. Verlangieri theorizes that vitamin C deficiency causes atherosclerosis. True, cholesterol does clog arteries. But in Dr. Verlangieri's view, cholesterol is really a Johnny-come-lately, a cardiovascular bad guy who takes advantage of an already bad situation caused by a vitamin C deficiency.

One study by Dr. Verlangieri and his colleagues at the University of Mississippi lends support to his controversial theory of vitamin C's role.

Dr. Verlangieri and his staff reviewed health statistics from the period between 1964 and 1978. During that time, he noticed, Americans increased their intake of fruits and vegetables rich in vitamin C. Deaths from cardiovascular disease during that period declined.

Other experts also have noted the decline in cardiovascular deaths and have attributed the slide to a number of factors, including a reduction in smoking, better eating habits and an increase in physical activity. But in his study, Dr. Verlangieri credited the increased intake of foods rich in vitamin C for the decline in heart deaths.

According to Dr. Verlangieri's research, vitamin C turns off an enzyme that attacks what are called endothelial cells in blood vessel walls. If you are vitamin C deficient—that is, if your cells aren't saturated with vitamin C—the enzyme is free to do its dirty work.

"The cells of blood vessels can be compared to bricks in a wall," explains Dr. Verlangieri. "Mortar holds the bricks in the wall together, but in blood vessels, a cement called the extracellular matrix holds the cells together. If the cement becomes defective, the cells loosen up. That leaves some bare spots. Normally, the cells provide a barrier to keep cholesterol off the blood vessel walls. But when the cholesterol gets into those bare spots, it causes inflammation. Vitamin C actually works at the level of the cell to inhibit an enzyme that chews up that cement."

If the body is low in vitamin C, the blood vessel walls become denuded in spots, says Dr. Verlangieri, leaving convenient places for cholesterol to take root. So cholesterol is an important part of the process once the disease begins, but it isn't how the disease begins.

If the theory is true, how much vitamin C would people need to prevent cardiovascular disease? According to Dr. Verlangieri, the Recommended Dietary Allowance (RDA) of 60 milligrams isn't enough. "I think the evidence suggests that from 1,000 to 2,000 milligrams is probably what we need," he says.

Not a Do-It-Yourself Treatment

Before you consider increasing your intake of C, bear in mind that in many quarters this theory is still controversial. Many scientists do not think vitamin C is involved in coronary artery disease. Others do believe vitamin C appears to reduce coronary risks, but for altogether different reasons.

One study, for instance, suggests vitamin C in 1,000-milligram doses prevents blood platelets from clumping together and adhering to blood vessel walls. To find out whether this is true, researchers at

Best Food Sources of Vitamin C

Food	Portion	Vitamin C (mg.)
Orange juice, freshly squeezed	1 cup	124
Grapefruit juice, freshly squeezed	1 cup	94
Papaya	½ medium	94
Guava	½	83
Kiwifruit	1 medium	75
Orange	1	70
Brussels sprouts, raw	4	65
Green peppers, raw, chopped	½ cup	64
Cantaloupe	¼	56
Watermelon	¹⁄₁₆	47
Tomato juice	1 cup	45
Strawberries	½ cup	42
Broccoli, raw, chopped	½ cup	41
Grapefruit	½	39
Cauliflower, raw, chopped	½ cup	36
Potato, baked	1 medium	26
Tangerine	1	26
Tomato, raw	1	22
Lemon	1 wedge	21
Turnip greens, cooked, chopped	½ cup	20
Cabbage, raw, chopped	½ cup	17
Blackberries	½ cup	15
Raspberries	½ cup	15
Banana	1	11
Blueberries	½ cup	9
Spinach, raw, chopped	½ cup	8
Snap beans, green, boiled	½ cup	6
Cherries, sweet	½ cup	5
Mung bean sprouts	¼ cup	3

SOURCES: Adapted from Agriculture Handbook Nos. 8-9, 8-11 (Washington, D.C.: U.S. Department of Agriculture).

Tagore Medical College and Hospital in India gave volunteers 1,000 milligrams of vitamin C every eight hours for ten days. At the end of that period, they drew blood samples and found a significant drop in the rate at which blood platelets clumped together and adhered.

But at the same time, researchers noted that they were administering vitamin C in "pharmacologic doses"—doses so high they should be taken only under a doctor's supervision. They concluded that further studies needed to be done to confirm their findings. But whatever the connection, research at least suggests that there might be one.

Make This Your D-Day

He was certain he was about to die. At 82, the infirmities of old age had been limited to a mild case of diabetes and a hip fracture, from which he had recently recovered. Now he found himself back in the hospital, his bones weak and aching from what he was sure was an insidious cancer eating him alive.

Fortunately, his doctor's diagnosis wasn't made in such terrified haste. In fact, this physician even refused to jump to an easy conclusion when the x-rays showed the classic symptoms of osteoporosis: a wasting of bone mass and many collapsed vertebrae. His decision to prescribe vitamin D and calcium was based in part on something his frightened elderly patient told him in conversation: that he avoided sunlight and didn't drink milk or take vitamins.

Uriel A. Barzel, M.D., of New York City's Montefiore Medical Group and Albert Einstein School of Medicine, suspected that what he was seeing, x-rays and patient's fears aside, was osteomalacia, an adult version of a now rare childhood disease called rickets, which is a result of vitamin D deficiency. Both conditions are characterized by painful, thinning bones that, left untreated, can lead to deformities.

New Healing Possibilities for Vitamin D

Vitamin D is converted by the liver and kidneys into its active form, a hormone called calcitriol that regulates the calcium balance in the body. Research in Japan has found that the hormone suppresses leukemia cells by causing them to be turned into noncancerous cells.

"Where this will go therapeutically isn't clear at this stage," says Hector DeLuca, Ph.D., professor of biochemistry at the University of Wisconsin, Madison. "In the long run, someday we may be able to control some types of leukemia. This may also have applications for controlling other types of malignancies."

Dr. DeLuca's own research also suggests that a vitamin D deficiency may lead to problems with glucose metabolism and, ultimately, insulin secretion. "Part of the falloff in glucose tolerance that occurs in many older people could be due to a lack of vitamin D, so if we can prevent the deficiency of calcitriol, perhaps we can control some cases of diabetes."

There's also a chance that a form of hearing loss associated

Until recent years, vitamin D deficiency was thought to be almost as rare as the bubonic plague, eradicated by vitamin D-fortified foods such as milk. But in the past few years, researchers and clinicians alike have become concerned that it may be a serious hidden problem among the nation's elderly. One researcher calls it "an unrecognized epidemic," and it may be implicated as a factor in that scourge of old age, hip fracture. What's more, it's often difficult to diagnose, frequently masquerading as that other bone-thinning condition, osteoporosis.

Dr. Barzel took an educated guess with his patient and was proved correct in the best possible way—the man got well after three weeks of treatment with supplements. But, Dr. Barzel acknowledges, osteomalacia is a diagnosis that's easy to miss.

with the cochlea, a tube shaped like a snail shell that forms a crucial part of the inner ear, can be prevented. Apparently, the cochlea needs vitamin D and calcium just as much as the skeleton and teeth do. When a deficiency occurs, minerals and hearing slowly fade. So far, hearing has been restored in some cases with daily supplements of calcium and vitamin D.

Preventing the hearing condition or catching it in the early phase is essential, since the deafness may be reversible. Just as important is the fact that early detection could point to the onset of bone-degenerating osteomalacia before more serious skeletal problems occur.

As if the case for getting out in the sunshine weren't strong enough, a study spanning almost two decades found that men who developed colorectal cancer had lower intakes of vitamin D and calcium. A research team of scientists from across the country discovered that those men who developed cancer also weighed more and got less exercise than those who remained free of the disease, which, according to the researchers, "supports the suggestion that physical activity is inversely associated with the risk of colon cancer."

A Disease in Disguise

"Because vitamin D deficiency is uncommon in the general population, the family physician or internist may fail to consider vitamin D and may miss this diagnosis in the elderly," the physician says. "The symptoms and signs of early vitamin D deficiency may be difficult to recognize. The patient may have weakness, which may be attributed to coexisting disease. Although bone pain is quite specific, it may be mistaken for metastatic disease [cancer] or osteoporosis not only by the patient but also by the physician."

Although a bone biopsy may tell the most accurate story, Dr. Barzel has advised other physicians to first ask the right questions to pinpoint whether a patient is getting an adequate amount of vitamin D. If not, a short therapeutic trial with moderate amounts of vitamin D and calcium can be diagnosis and cure in one. "The response of the patient is both quick and dramatic and confirms the diagnosis," Dr. Barzel says.

Better diagnostic techniques are imperative because a number of studies give every indication that vitamin D deficiency is not rare. In fact, there may be cause for alarm. Studies of health-conscious and apparently healthy elderly participants showed that at least half got less than the minimum daily requirement of vitamin D—200 international units. A third were getting less than 100 international units. In a study of 142 elderly hip fracture patients at Massachusetts General Hospital in Boston, 40 percent were vitamin D deficient and three-quarters of them had osteomalacia. "As many as 30 to 40 percent of all hip fracture patients in the United States have osteomalacia," says researcher Samuel H. Doppelt, M.D., assistant professor of orthopaedic surgery and medicine at Harvard Medical School.

How Vitamin D Works

To understand these figures, it's first necessary to understand how vitamin D works. In the body, the raw vitamin is changed into its active form, a hormone known as calcitriol, by the kidneys and the liver. This active form enhances the absorption of calcium to nourish the nerves, muscles and skeleton. Without vitamin D, the body begins to strip-mine the bones for calcium to meet the needs of the nerves and muscles, leaving the bones thin, brittle and breakable.

In its advanced stages, osteomalacia can be extremely painful and may be accompanied by tetany, muscle spasms that are caused by a calcium imbalance. But even before pain starts, a deficiency of vitamin D can do enough damage to cripple. It is a hidden epidemic in many ways. "A vitamin D deficiency of less severity can cause an accumulated bone loss with age and can be painless until a bone break occurs," says A. Michael Parfitt, M.D., director of the Bone and Mineral Research Laboratory at Henry Ford Hospital in Detroit. "And I'm afraid this is rather common among elderly people."

The reason? Although it is difficult for most of us to avoid getting enough vitamin D, it's even more difficult for elderly people to get enough. It's abundant only in foods that are hardly a staple of the

American menu: fatty fish such as mackerel and swordfish. (See the table on page 54.) In the United States, vitamin D is added to milk, which many elderly people use simply to color tea or coffee. But it's most abundantly supplied when the sun's ultraviolet rays strike the skin, activating a vitamin D precursor. About 90 percent of the major circulating form of vitamin D comes from our skin supply. In fact, basking in the sun for about 15 to 30 minutes a day is enough to eliminate the need for any dietary vitamin D at all in healthy adults.

Older Skin Needs Its Day in the Sun

Researchers aren't sure why, but the skin of young people appears to be a more efficient vitamin D factory than the skin of older adults. As skin ages and becomes thinner, it becomes less productive at turning out vitamin D from sunlight, according to one study.

To prove the point, scientists took skin samples from a number of surgical patients. The patients ranged in age from 8 to 92. Each sample

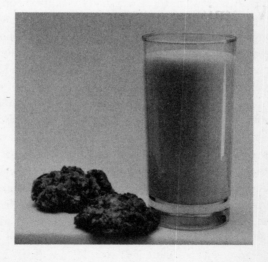

Vitamin D is essential for calcium absorption from food; without it the body begins to pilfer calcium from the bones, weakening them and causing deformities. Drinking fortified milk is one of the most reliable ways to ensure an adequate supply of vitamin D.

was bathed in ultraviolet light—similar to the ultraviolet light in sunlight. When they checked the samples, they found that young skin produced the most vitamin D. In the older, thinner skin samples, vitamin D production decreased in proportion to the age of the individual. The skin of one 82-year-old produced less than half the amount of vitamin D churned out by the 8-year-old skin.

Like Dr. Barzel's patient, however, many elderly people don't get enough sun. They may be housebound by illness or disability, or simply less physically active and less likely to spend time outdoors. But, for whatever reason, they simply don't tap into the most available supply of vitamin D there is.

Theoretically, doctors could solve the problem by prescribing cruises to warm, sunny islands or, at the very least, daily strolls in the afternoon sun. A group of British doctors stopped just short of recommending that when they assessed the vitamin D status of 110 men and women nearing retirement age. They extolled the virtues of "a sunny holiday" when they saw what it did to the vitamin D levels of their subjects. Almost all of those who had the highest concentrations of circulating vitamin D had been on vacation in sunnier climates, some as long as four months previously. One woman, whose diet was relatively poor in vitamin D, nevertheless had the highest concentration of the vitamin D in her bloodstream. The reason? She had just gotten a two-week dose of sunshine on Malta.

But for many, a vacation in the sun simply isn't possible. And the sun isn't always an entirely reliable source of the sunshine vitamin either. During the winter months, the sun slants its rays through the ozone layer of the atmosphere, which filters out much of the ultraviolet light the skin needs to manufacture vitamin D. Studies show that blood levels of the vitamin tend to drop in the winter, especially among elderly women. Urban dwellers may see the sun even less than the housebound, especially if they live and work in the shadows of tall buildings. Pollution may also be a factor. A progressive increase in atmospheric ozone and pollutants between 1951 and 1972 produced a 20 percent decrease in the amount of ultraviolet radiation reaching the earth. Some researchers believe the decrease in ultraviolet light parallels a progressive increase in hip fracture mortality.

How much sunlight does older skin need to make enough vitamin D?

Vegetarians Need Vitamin D, Too

The elderly aren't the only people who need vitamin D. Everyone needs vitamin D for strong bones, but not everyone gets enough. Among the most vulnerable are vegetarians, whose diets don't always provide sufficient vitamin D. Additionally, the high percentage of roughage in a vegetarian's diet may interfere with the absorption of this important vitamin.

Consider, for example, the severe deficiencies reported by researchers in Norway among vegetarian children. Several children in that country were hospitalized for rickets, or osteomalacia, a disease characterized by progressive bone softening.

These children also may have been predisposed to rickets because of the vitamin D-deficient diets of their vegetarian mothers, according to researchers.

After they were diagnosed, the children were given vitamin D supplements, and the painful symptoms of rickets disappeared altogether.

"That is almost impossible to say precisely," says Michael F. Holick, M.D., Ph.D., director of the Vitamin D and Bone Metabolism Laboratory at Tufts University in Massachusetts. "It depends on so many things—skin pigmentation, time of year, location and so on. But we can say this: If, say, you're in Boston in June at noontime, you should expose your hands, face and arms, 15 minutes at a time. In the winter, you'd probably have to expose a much larger area of the skin for a much longer period of time because the sun's rays are much weaker [and even that may be insufficient]. In this case, vitamin D supplements are a desirable alternative," he says.

Faulty Metabolism Can Cause Trouble

There is another confounding factor. Elderly people also may have faulty vitamin D metabolism—an inability to convert vitamin D into

Best Food Sources of Vitamin D

Food	Portion	Vitamin D (I.U.)
Halibut-liver oil	2 tsp.	9,636
Herring, grilled	3 oz.	850
Mackerel, fried	3 oz.	717
Cod-liver oil	2 tsp.	675
Mackerel, raw	3 oz.	595
Salmon, Pacific, steamed	3 oz.	425
Sardines, canned in oil, drained	3 oz.	255
Tuna, canned in oil, drained	3 oz.	197
Milk, 1% fat	1 cup	102

SOURCES: Adapted from *McCance and Widdowson's The Composition of Foods,* by A. A. Paul and D. A. T. Southgate (New York: Elsevier/North-Holland Biomedical, 1978).

its active form in adequate amounts. Hector DeLuca, Ph.D., professor of biochemistry at the University of Wisconsin, Madison, with his colleagues, was the first to demonstrate that vitamin D has to be changed into an active hormonal form before it can function. Since isolating the hormone, Dr. DeLuca and others have been experimenting with ways to use it pharmacologically to treat postmenopausal and old-age osteoporosis.

"In both old age and the postmenopausal state, the vitamin D hormone doesn't respond as it should," says Dr. DeLuca. "Calcium absorption is low; bone turnover—the tearing down of old bone and the rebuilding of new bone—is low. If you have low calcium absorption, the body continues to draw on bone calcium to meet nerve and muscle needs. This contributes to the thinning of bones. When they become thin enough, they fracture."

Several clinical tests have been "promising," says Dr. DeLuca.

Postmenopausal women given small doses of the vitamin D hormone had increased calcium retention in the bones, increased bone mass and a decrease in bone fracture rates. The hormone works, apparently, because it circumvents the metabolism problem. Giving vitamin D alone is ineffective, says Dr. DeLuca.

But if your metabolism is working up to par and you're in the high-risk category, a supplement may be needed. "Without vitamin D, you can't make the hormonal form," says the researcher. "I personally think the best way to get this vitamin is by sunlight. But, unlike some other nutrition people, I recommend a multivitamin so you can get all the basic nutrients you need, including vitamin D."

If you are taking a vitamin D supplement, make sure it's no more than 400 international units a day. Vitamin D in larger amounts can be toxic. "Taking 400 international units once a day will keep you well below the level that can cause any harm," says Dr. Parfitt.

The Best Calcium for Your Bones

Unless you've been doing time in a Tibetan monastery, you've probably heard reports of how important calcium is for healthy bones. It's the element that keeps us standing tall, even as we age.

You may know calcium's benefits, but do you know how much calcium you're actually getting? And how to get as much as you need? Dietitians say most people have little idea how much calcium is in the foods they eat. And that they're unlikely to know that the Recommended Dietary Allowance (RDA) is 800 milligrams for adults or that the National Institutes of Health recommend 1,000 milligrams daily for premenopausal women and 1,500 milligrams daily for postmenopausal women. Most people simply have no way of telling if their daily intake is adequate.

The following examples of types of people who may be at risk for calcium deficiency should help you to evaluate and, if necessary, correct your own diet. In many cases, simple changes in food choices are all that's needed. Where that's not possible, it's important to know how much additional calcium you may need as a supplement.

Perpetual Dieters

If you're trying to lose weight to improve your health, the last thing you want to do is cause a new health problem in the process.

"My experience is that people who are dieting are so wrapped up in losing weight that they don't pay attention to nutrient needs," says Patricia Hausman, nutritionist and author of *The Calcium Bible.* "They have to make a conscious effort if they are to get the calcium they need."

There are plenty of low-fat, low-calorie, calcium-rich foods. "If they have at least three glasses of skim milk a day, they're doing reasonably well," Hausman says. Each cup has about 300 milligrams of calcium. Or dieters can dig into bok choy, broccoli or kale, or collard, mustard or turnip greens. One cup of any of these vegetables (cooked) provides at least 100 milligrams of calcium and less than 50 calories.

Some cheeses are fairly low in calories. One ounce of mozzarella

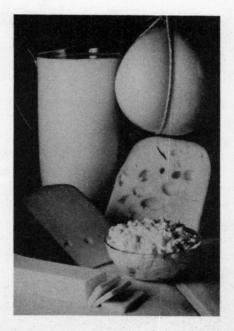

Skim milk and low-fat cheeses are available to help people who are concerned about cutting down on dietary fat and cholesterol get their fair share of calcium from dairy foods.

or provolone has more than 100 milligrams of calcium and about 100 calories. A half cup of 1 percent fat cottage cheese has 70 milligrams of calcium and 82 calories. The same amount of part-skim ricotta has 340 milligrams of calcium. Unfortunately, it also has 171 calories. A cup of nonfat yogurt has 450 milligrams of calcium and 125 calories. Canned salmon (be sure to eat those soft little bones!), shrimp and oysters are also delicious, low-calorie sources of calcium.

If you find that your diet simply isn't adding up, and you're not willing to make the dietary changes that boost calcium, consider adding supplements. The most common forms are calcium carbonate, calcium lactate, calcium gluconate, dicalcium phosphate and oyster shell (basically calcium carbonate). Current evidence suggests that most people absorb each of these equally well.

Look for the number of milligrams of calcium per tablet. Some supplements have relatively little calcium, making them an impractical source. Calcium carbonate has the highest concentration of calcium, followed by calcium phosphate, then calcium lactate. Consider the

---

Quick Calcium Calculations

Here's a simple way to determine how much calcium you're getting from food.

Any one of the following will give you about 300 milligrams or more of calcium: 8 ounces of skim, low-fat or whole milk or buttermilk; 1½ ounces of hard cheese; one cup of yogurt; 1½ slices of processed cheese; two cups of cottage cheese; two cups of ice milk or ice cream; 3 to 4 ounces of salmon (with bones); 3 ounces of sardines (with bones); 3 ounces of tofu (made with a calcium coagulant).

For a rough estimate of your daily intake, figure that three to four servings a day of any of these foods will put you into the 900- to 1,200-milligram range. The Recommended Dietary Allowance for calcium is 800 milligrams, although it's suggested that women get 1,000 to 1,500 milligrams a day to ward off osteoporosis.

number of tablets you have to take to meet your daily quota. It's easier to take two or three than eight or ten.

Milk-Shunning Adults

Mom's no longer there to coax you to drain that glass, so perhaps milk's no longer on your menu, except in coffee or tea. For adults, and, for that matter, kids who won't drink milk, calcium intake is likely to be precariously low. Other food sources normally provide only 200 to 300 milligrams of calcium a day.

If milk just isn't your cup of tea, try disguising its taste, suggests Hausman. Use plenty of milk in pancakes, cereals, shakes and puddings. Add powdered milk to everything from creamy salad dressings to meat

---

How to Have a Calcium-Rich Day

As this typical day's menu shows, there are easy, delicious ways to incorporate this important mineral into every meal. The foods in this menu provide a total of 1,251 milligrams of calcium.

Breakfast

1 cup plain low-fat yogurt (415 milligrams) with ½ banana
   and 1 tablespoon wheat germ
1 cup orange juice
   Tea with lemon and honey

Lunch

1 ounce Monterey Jack cheese (212 milligrams) melted on
   whole wheat bread, with lettuce and tomato
1 cup cream of asparagus soup (175 milligrams)
1 cup apricot juice

Dinner

3 ounces canned salmon with bones (271 milligrams), served
   over pasta with spicy, chunky tomato sauce
1 cup cooked broccoli (178 milligrams)
1 cup apple crisp

loaf. And make sure you're getting at least three servings a day of cheese, yogurt (try frozen soft-serve yogurt for a treat) or high-calcium nondairy foods, like sardines, oysters or shrimp.

If milk or other dairy products cause diarrhea and gas, you may be lactose intolerant. You lack an enzyme that allows your bowel to break down milk sugars. But that doesn't mean dairy products are entirely off-limits. Look for brands of milk in which the lactose has already been broken down, or add a powdered enzyme, available at drugstores, to your regular brand. Try yogurt, which has less lactose than milk, provided it has no added milk solids.

Some people with lactose intolerance can eat some dairy products without symptoms, and they usually have fewer symptoms if they mix dairy products with other foods. Lactose intolerance does not significantly impair your ability to absorb calcium.

Growing Teenagers

If you've got one, you know that teenagers are notorious for eating exactly what they want. And what they prefer usually comes in a bag from a drive-through window.

"Some fast foods can be good sources of calcium," says Ellen Coleman, a registered dietitian at the Riverside Cardiac Fitness Center in Riverside, California. The average fast-food cheeseburger provides 150 milligrams of calcium; one-fourth of a 14-inch pizza, 290 milligrams; a taco with cheese, 110 milligrams; a ten-ounce vanilla shake, 325 milligrams.

Of course, these aren't foods you'd want to eat every day. "They have too much fat and too many calories for the amount of nutrients they deliver," Coleman says. She finds that most teenagers, when invited to indulge, also consume large quantities of calcium-rich chocolate milk, frozen yogurt, puddings, custards, cream soups, soufflés and cheese sauces.

The calcium RDA for ages 11 to 18 is 1,200 milligrams. That's as high as it is for pregnant women. And it's a level few teenagers seem to achieve. That concerns some bone-metabolism specialists, who say the best time to increase bone mass is before age 35. Scrimping on calcium during adolescence may be the perfect setup for osteoporosis later in life.

People with Low Stomach Acid

As they age, many people experience decreased stomach acidity. They probably won't have much trouble absorbing calcium from the foods they eat, since the food itself stimulates stomach acid production. But they may have problems taking in the calcium from supplements, especially on an empty stomach. Some acid is needed to absorb calcium carbonate, but an empty stomach usually contains none.

"It might be a good idea for older people and those with known impairment of gastric acid secretion to take their calcium supplement with meals," says Robert Recker, M.D., of the Creighton University School of Medicine, Omaha, Nebraska. Dr. Recker has found that the presence of a meal in the stomach is sufficient to permit normal absorption of calcium carbonate, even in patients with low stomach acid.

Or they might want to consider switching to calcium citrate, a water-soluble form of calcium. Dr. Recker found that when people with low stomach acid took their calcium without food, they absorbed only 5 percent of calcium carbonate. In contrast, they absorbed 45 percent of calcium citrate.

Kidney-Stone Formers

Almost everyone can safely consume up to 1,200 milligrams of calcium a day. "People who form kidney stones, though, shouldn't be taking calcium supplements without a doctor's supervision," says Charles Pak, M.D., chief of mineral metabolism at the University of Texas Health Science Center, Dallas. "In stone formers, calcium supplements lead to excessive calcium levels in the urine, which can aggravate stone formation."

Stone formers who want to take supplemental calcium might try calcium citrate, Dr. Pak says. This compound increases levels of urinary citrate, a substance that inhibits formation of calcium stones.

Pregnant and Lactating Women

Because estrogen levels are high during pregnancy, you have the potential for building bone tissue, provided you get plenty of calcium. Calcium demands are high during pregnancy—1,200 milligrams a day.

Best Food Sources of Calcium

Food	Portion	Calcium (mg.)
Tofu, raw, firm, coagulated with calcium sulfate	3 oz.	581
Swiss cheese	2 oz.	544
Provolone cheese	2 oz.	428
Monterey Jack cheese	2 oz.	424
Yogurt, low-fat	1 cup	415
Cheddar cheese	2 oz.	408
Muenster cheese	2 oz.	406
Colby cheese	2 oz.	388
Brick cheese	2 oz.	382
Sardines, Atlantic, drained	3 oz.	372
American cheese	2 oz.	348
Ricotta cheese, part-skim	½ cup	337
Milk, skim	1 cup	302
Mozzarella cheese	2 oz.	294
Milk, whole	1 cup	291
Buttermilk	1 cup	285
Limburger cheese	2 oz.	282
Ice milk, soft-serve	1 cup	274
Salmon, sockeye, drained	3 oz.	271
Ice cream	1 cup	176
Ice milk	1 cup	176

Most prenatal supplements don't provide much of the mineral, Coleman says. And obstetricians don't always pay calcium the attention it deserves. It may be up to you to beef up your diet to get enough, or to tell your doctor you want to take supplemental calcium. Calcium needs are even higher during breastfeeding than during pregnancy, although the RDA is the same, Hausman says. "A woman who breastfeeds her baby for nine months loses three to four times as much calcium in her milk as she lost during her nine months of pregnancy."

Food	Portion	Calcium (mg.)
Tofu, raw, firm, coagulated with nigari	3 oz.	174
Pizza, cheese	⅛ of 14″ pie	144
Blackstrap molasses	1 tbsp.	137
Almonds	¼ cup	100
Scallops, steamed	3 oz.	98
Broccoli, cooked	½ cup	89
Soybeans, cooked	½ cup	88
Parmesan cheese	1 tbsp.	86
Collards, cooked	½ cup	74
Dandelion greens, cooked	½ cup	74
Navy beans, cooked	½ cup	64
Soy flour, defatted	¼ cup	60
Shrimp, raw	3 oz.	54
Mustard greens, cooked	½ cup	52
Kale, cooked	½ cup	47
Broccoli, raw	1 cup	42

SOURCES: Adapted from
Agriculture Handbook Nos. 8, 8-1, 456 (Washington, D.C.: U.S. Department of Agriculture).
Nutrient Data Research Branch, U.S. Department of Agriculture, Washington, D.C.

Athletes

It's true that physical activity helps keep your bones strong. But exercise by itself is not enough. You need calcium, too.

And too much physical activity can actually hurt bones. Women runners who have stopped menstruating experience a rapid loss of calcium from the bones, probably because of a drop in estrogen levels. They need to train less and eat more, especially calcium-rich dairy foods.

Rate Your Iron Reserves

When it comes to your health, iron is a metal more precious than gold.

Although you may hoard it like a miser—banking the iron from a weekly serving of liver, a daily iron supplement and plates full of spinach and broccoli—your account may be regularly depleted by the iron robbers. If you are a menstruating woman, a dieter, a vegetarian, even a heavy tea drinker, you can find yourself overdrawn at the iron bank despite all your good intentions. In fact, you could be making withdrawals as fast as you're making deposits.

When that happens, your energy stores go bankrupt. Even before you're in the throes of fullblown anemia, you may experience fatigue, dizziness, nausea, loss of appetite and a shortened attention span.

Are You Food Rich but Iron Poor?

How do you rate your iron levels? It's much like auditing any other account. First, you start by looking in the deposit column.

Part I of this quick and easy quiz will let you know roughly whether your weekly menu is iron rich or iron poor. It won't tell you if you're meeting the Recommended Dietary Allowance (10 milligrams daily for men, 18 milligrams for women). It's not that precise. But it will give you some idea of what kind of an iron-saver you are.

But the total of your deposits means nothing until you fill in the withdrawal column, Part II of the quiz. These are the risk factors, each one eager to pocket your savings of this most precious metal. Needless to say, if your Part II total equals or exceeds the total from Part I (+16, −19, for example), you may have to make some dietary or life-style changes to avoid the penalties of iron deficiency. If your Part I score is low, yet still higher than your score for Part II (+9, −7, for example), you are probably not getting many iron-rich foods in your diet, and consequently you may not be getting enough iron despite your low risk-factor score. If the scores are close (+15, −14, for example), you may still want to make some life-style or dietary changes that will shrink your withdrawals and boost your deposits.

Now take the following quiz, calculate *two* totals (don't add them), and compare. Then read the explanation of what it all means to your health.

Test Your Iron Levels

Part I: Deposits

1. Do you eat beef liver at least once a week?   +3 points   _____

2. Do you eat a portion of beef, turkey, chicken, fish or shellfish at least once a day?   +3 points   _____

3. If you answered no to question 2, do you eat a portion of beef, turkey, chicken, fish or shellfish two to four times a week?   +1 point   _____

Bonus: Give yourself   +3 points if you eat meat for three meals a day.   _____

4. Does your diet include a serving of blackstrap molasses, almonds, lima beans, peas, sunflower seeds, prunes, dried apricots or broccoli at least twice a week?   +2 points   _____

Answer the next five questions and bonus questions only if you answered yes to any of the previous questions.

5. Does your diet include a serving of orange juice, green peppers, grapefruit juice, papaya, brussels sprouts, oranges, turnip

greens, cantaloupe, cauliflower, strawberries, tomato juice, grapefruit, potatoes, raw tomatoes, cabbage, blackberries, blueberries or cherries at least twice a week?   +2 points   _____

6. Does your diet include a serving of organ meats, yogurt, almonds, wild rice, ricotta cheese, Swiss cheese, Camembert cheese or Roquefort cheese at least twice a week?   +2 points   _____

7. Does your diet include a serving of cashews, mushrooms, pecans, bananas, walnuts, peanuts, wheat germ, prunes or sesame seeds at least twice a week?   +2 points   _____

Bonus: Give yourself +1 point each if your diet frequently includes broccoli, dried apricots or almonds.   _____

Give yourself +½ point each if your diet frequently includes brussels sprouts, cauliflower, peas, bananas, strawberries, cashews, sunflower seeds, chicken, chicken livers or brewer's yeast.   _____

8. Do you take a B-complex or riboflavin supplement (no score for multivitamins)?   +2 points   _____

9. Do you take vitamin C supplements?   +2 points   _____

10. Do you take an iron supplement?   +3 points   _____

11. Does your typical meal include meat, a vegetable and one of the following: orange juice, green peppers, grapefruit juice, papaya, brussels sprouts, broccoli, oranges, turnip greens, cantaloupe, cauliflower, strawberries, tomato juice, grapefruit, potatoes, tomatoes, cabbage, blackberries, blueberries or cherries?   +3 points   _____

12. Do you frequently use iron cookware?   +3 points   _____

Part I Total   _____

Part II: Withdrawals

1. Are you a menstruating woman?   −3 points   _____

2. Do you have heavy menstrual flow?   −3 points   _____

3. If you are a woman, do you give blood twice or more a year?   −2 points   _____

4. Have you recently had surgery?   −3 points   _____

5. Do you have a peptic ulcer, colitis or hemorrhoids?   −3 points   _____

6. Do you take aspirin often?   −2 points   _____

7. Are you on a low-calorie diet?   −3 points   _____

8. Are you over 65?   −3 points   _____

9. Do you drink a lot of tea, especially during or after meals?   −3 points   _____

10. Do you eat a lot of foods containing the preservative EDTA and phosphate additives?   −3 points   _____

11. Do you drink a lot of coffee, especially during and after meals?   −2 points   _____

12. Do you eat a high-fiber diet?   −½ point   _____

13. Are you a vegetarian?   −2 points   _____

14. Do you take calcium supplements?   −½ point   _____

15. Do you frequently take antacids?   −½ point   _____

16. Do you live in an area exposed to industrial pollution, particularly cadmium and lead?   −1 point   _____

17. Are you involved in strenuous activity, such as long-distance running?   −1 point   _____

18. Do you feel you are under a great deal of stress?   −2 points   _____

Part II Total   _____

Explanation

Part I: Deposits

1. Beef liver is one of the best sources of dietary iron, containing 5.3 milligrams per three-ounce serving. That doesn't mean your body can absorb the total amount. Only about 25 percent of the iron from animal sources is bioavailable—that is, absorbed by the body. Some medical experts believe many iron deficiency problems are the result of poor bioavailability rather than low iron intake. That's why beef liver is so important: It gets high scores not only for iron content but also for bioavailability.

In fact, you'd have to eat about 14 pounds of broccoli to get the amount of iron absorbed from six to seven ounces of liver. And there's a bonus, too. Liver also contains three other important nutrients: vitamin C, riboflavin and copper, all of which enhance the absorption of iron.

2-3. Again, only meat and fish have that double whammy, high iron and high bioavailability. Though red meat is highest on both counts, both poultry and fish are good substitutes. Three ounces of dark-meat turkey contain two milligrams of iron; a three-ounce slice of light-meat chicken provides 0.9 milligrams, but it also contains the enhancer riboflavin, which increases iron bioavailability. And if you choose lean cuts of meat, you can keep calorie and cholesterol levels down near those of fish and poultry.

Bonus: Not only do you get a hefty dose of iron from meat, but its presence in a meal will help you absorb iron from other foods you're eating. You can increase your iron intake by spreading out your meat protein—not necessarily increasing the amount you eat—over three meals instead of one or two.

4. If you don't eat meat, and even if you do, you might want to consider including as many of these foods in your diet as possible. They're all iron rich, but only about 5 percent of the iron they contain is bioavailable.

But there are ways to increase bioavailability. Take a look at the foods listed in questions 5, 6 and 7 and the bonus question. If you can design your menu around these foods, you can sometimes double or triple iron absorption from both animal and plant sources.

5. The foods listed in this question are high in vitamin C. In one study done at the University of Göteborg, in Sweden, a glass of orange juice served with a meal of hamburger, string beans and mashed potatoes increased iron absorption from the meal by 85 percent. The same researchers were also able to significantly boost the iron absorption from a vegetarian meal by making sure it had a high vitamin C content.

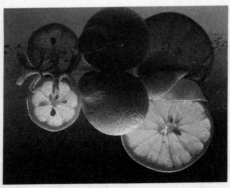

It's common knowledge that citrus fruits such as oranges and lemons are high in vitamin C, which is essential for many reasons. One of the most important may be that vitamin C makes it easier for the body to absorb iron, a nutrient that's vital for maintaining high energy levels.

6-7. These are the high-riboflavin and high-copper foods, respectively. Again, they're the helper nutrients that make sure you get the most out of your iron deposits.

Bonus: Why extra points for these foods? Broccoli, dried apricots and almonds contain not only iron but also at least two iron enhancers. The foods in the second bonus list contain iron and at least one enhancer nutrient.

8-10. Needless to say, taking supplements of iron and the enhancer nutrients can help if you can't eat enough to boost your iron savings.

11. You may recognize this food list. These are the vitamin C foods, and this is the ideal iron-rich meal: meat, iron-rich vegetable and vitamin C food.

12. Iron pans for iron nutrition? It sounds farfetched, but it really helps. The cooking process permits a considerable amount of iron to be absorbed by the food. In some cases, food cooked in iron cookware can have three or four times more iron than the same foods cooked in aluminum or glass. If you do a lot of wok cooking, you can bring up your deposit score.

Part II: Withdrawals

1-6. A government survey estimated that about 93 percent of all American women eat less than the Recommended Dietary Allowance of iron. That's the first strike against women. The second is blood loss from menstruation.

Iron is used by the body to form hemoglobin in the blood to help circulate oxygen and carbon dioxide. Because of its presence in the blood, any blood loss—from menstruation, surgery, ulcers, colitis, hemorrhoids, blood donations, even minor bleeding caused by aspirin—can leach iron from your system. Though men can certainly undergo surgery, have colitis or take aspirin, they're not as vulnerable as women. Why? Because menstruation, especially heavy menstruation (such as that caused by intrauterine devices), is a regular, monthly blood loss. It's an iron withdrawal women can, unfortunately, count on. That's why the Recommended Dietary Allowance for women is almost twice that for men. And women also often face a third strike: a low-calorie (and often low-meat) diet.

7. Even when women aren't dieting, they simply do not eat as many calories as men, and their intake of red meat and liver is lower.

Some researchers believe they would have to eat at least as much as men to get that precious 18 milligrams of iron a day.

8. Here's another rub for women. When menopause hits, it becomes much easier for a woman to get enough iron. But menopause means you're getting older, and studies have shown the risk of iron deficiency increases with age for both men and women.

9. Drinking a cup of tea with a meal, even a meal containing a large quantity of meat and vitamin C, can reduce your iron absorption by one-half to almost two-thirds, according to several studies. Why? Researchers believe it's the tannic acid in tea that binds to the iron in the meal and makes it impossible for the body to absorb it. There are a number of other iron inhibitors.

10. The common additives EDTA and phosphates, which are added to soft drinks, baked goods and other foods, can prevent iron from being absorbed.

11. Though not as potent as tea, coffee taken during or after a meal can decrease iron absorption by about 39 percent.

12. Diets high in fiber can also inhibit iron absorption, so if you're taking an iron supplement, it would be best to take it well before meals.

13. Because the most bioavailable iron is in meat, vegetarians have a harder time getting the iron they need. More careful diet management—assembling a menu rich in iron-containing vegetables and nutrient enhancers—as well as supplementation might be in order for these individuals.

14. Inorganic calcium can be a potent iron blocker. Researchers have also looked at dairy products that are high in calcium, but there's no clear evidence available to include them in the risk-factor category.

15. Why antacids? They can decrease the ability of gastric juices in the body to dissolve dietary iron.

16. Cadmium and lead, common industrial pollutants, are known iron inhibitors.

17. Strenuous exercise can rob you of iron. So-called sports anemia is relatively rare and may, in fact, be more related to diet than to exercise. Unless you are a very active person eating a low-calorie, iron-poor diet, you probably do not have to worry about this risk factor.

18. Stress robs us of so many things, it should be no surprise that iron is among them.

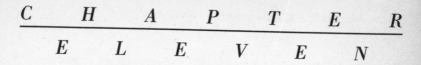

CHAPTER
ELEVEN

The Health Power of Magnesium

Everybody needs it, some owe their lives to it and doctors are starting to give it serious attention—magnesium is a little mineral with a big future. And the main reason is that scientific evidence on the health benefits of this mineral is coming in too fast to ignore.

Here's a rundown on further developments in this research.

Angina Attacks Stopped Cold

Following in the footsteps of other scientists, researchers in Israel have successfully treated 15 people afflicted with recurring spasm angina. At each bout of chest pains, the doctors injected the patients with magnesium. And 30 seconds to 5 minutes later, the attacks ceased. Ordinarily such attacks would last 5 to 15 minutes.

After these scientists demonstrated that they could use magnesium in angina treatment, they set out to test the mineral in angina prevention. They found that in several patients they could consistently provoke an angina attack by immersing the patients' hands in cold water. But if they injected the patients with magnesium before immersion, no attacks occurred. Magnesium apparently stopped the chest pains before they got started.

The results of these and other studies suggest that magnesium may one day replace or complement drugs as therapy for angina.

Diabetic Seizures Vanish

It's well established that intravenous magnesium is an anticonvulsant (agent for preventing or relieving convulsions) and that people with magnesium deficiencies sometimes suffer convulsions and tremors.

Doctors at the Bronx-Lebanon Hospital Center in the Bronx, New York, have used magnesium to stop seizures in people who have uncontrolled diabetes mellitus.

The seizures—marked by convulsive muscle contractions and jerky movements—afflicted three women with the disease. When the women were admitted to the hospital, their seizures were lasting from 30 seconds to three minutes, occurring every five to ten minutes. The doctors treated the patients' diabetes, but the seizures wouldn't stop. Since the physicians knew that magnesium deficiency is common in people with severe diabetes mellitus, they decided to inject the women with the mineral—and the injections worked. The seizures vanished within 24 hours after starting magnesium therapy.

"It therefore appears," the doctors report, "that magnesium deficiency was the main cause of the neuromuscular abnormality."

These results will have to be confirmed by additional research. But they do suggest an intriguing question: Can magnesium quell other kinds of seizures, including epileptic ones? Scientists surely will try to find out.

Heart Attack Damage Reduced

Research in both animals and people has hinted that magnesium may do "damage control" work during a heart attack, lessening the destruction of vital heart tissue.

Sherman Bloom, M.D., of George Washington University School of Medicine in Washington, D.C., has confirmed the earlier investigations. In a study focusing on heart attacks in dogs, he discovered that the animals on a low-magnesium diet suffered twice as much heart damage after an attack as animals on diets with adequate magnesium.

"When people have heart attacks—and they can have them without even knowing it—the critical consideration is how much damage is done to the heart muscle," Dr. Bloom says. "Every increase in infarcted area [destroyed tissue] increases your chances of dying in the aftermath of an attack. My study and research done by others indicate that magnesium is one very important determinant of how much damage a heart attack does.

"The data suggest," says Dr. Bloom, "that dietary magnesium intake is an important determining factor in your ability to withstand a heart attack. You should ensure that you're getting adequate amounts of magnesium in your diet."

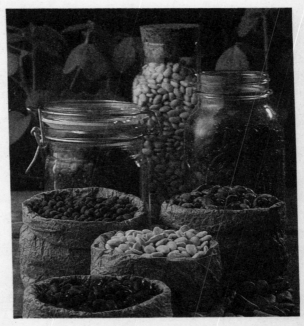

Lima beans, soybeans, kidney beans and black-eyed peas are all sources of magnesium, a mineral that, among other things, may help prevent high blood pressure in some people and reduce the severity of heart attack in others.

Type-A Behavior
and High Blood Pressure

The available evidence has suggested a compelling hypothesis: Type-A people (those who are hard-driving, impatient and excitable) react to stress by developing magnesium deficiencies, which in turn exaggerate the ill effects of stress and lead to high blood pressure.

Not too long ago, investigators in Paris reinforced the hypothesis when they studied 20 Type-A young men under stress.

When they gave these Type-A young men a stress-producing task to perform and monitored the magnesium in their bodies, the researchers uncovered an odd biochemical routine. Magnesium leached out of red blood cells and was shunted out of the body via the urine. This magnesium depletion happened in almost twice as many of the Type-A people as in a comparable group of more relaxed Type-B subjects.

"Type-A behavior personalities," says head researcher Jean-Georges Henrotte, M.D., "would be involved in a vicious circle in which their tendency to chronic self-induced stress would lead them to a progressively increasing state of magnesium deficiency."

And a lack of magnesium, as other research indicates, is probably a contributor to high blood pressure. Conversely, magnesium supplementation has actually been used to lower blood pressure.

"These results," says Dr. Henrotte, "should be, of course, confirmed on a larger group of individuals."

The Unhealthful Impact of Stress

Researchers have concluded that Type-A people may not be the only ones caught in a cycle of stress and magnesium deficiency. Studies have suggested that stress in almost anyone can deplete magnesium and that such depletion can magnify stress-induced ills.

Scientists at the University of Hohenheim in West Germany uncovered evidence that this stress/depletion cycle may be halted with magnesium supplements.

In studies of thousands of pigs subjected to the typical stresses of confinement, the researchers found that they could reduce the death rate of the animals by giving them extra magnesium. In fact, the death rates of supplemented pigs were one-seventh to one-half as high as the death rates of pigs getting normal levels of magnesium.

"These studies and others like them," says chief investigator Hans G. Classen, Ph.D., "indicate that with adequate magnesium stores, people may be better able to withstand the ravages of stress in their daily lives."

Irregular Heartbeat Normalized

Doctors have shown that magnesium may play a key role in the treatment of the potentially dangerous condition of arrhythmia, or irregular heartbeat.

Investigators at the University of California-Irvine College of Medicine corroborated the earlier evidence by using magnesium successfully to treat arrhythmia patients after standard therapies had failed.

"We've studied several patients with acute, life-threatening arrhythmias that wouldn't respond to either drugs or shock therapy," says chief researcher Lloyd T. Iseri, M.D. "But when the patients received magnesium, their heartbeats reverted to normal rhythm. The magnesium had an almost instant effect, whereas some drugs may take minutes to influence the arrhythmias."

It remains to be seen whether magnesium will become the therapy of choice in the treatment of arrhythmia.

Better Brain Function

Medical people have firmly documented the harm done to muscles and nerves by magnesium deficiency, but they know much less about what a lack of the mineral can do to the brain.

Paul G. Cohen, M.D., of Atlanta, reports that he's treated three adults suffering from brain disease and low magnesium levels. All three eventually lapsed into a coma. But when he gave them magnesium, they responded immediately. There was, Dr. Cohen says, "prompt reversal of encephalopathy [brain dysfunction] and coma."

Just how common are such symptoms in people lacking magnesium? How often is the magnesium connection overlooked? Future research and clinical experience will have to supply the answers.

Dossier on Magnesium

Here's an abbreviated report on magnesium: how much you need, who may be deficient and why it's necessary.

Recommended Dietary Allowance (RDA)

300 milligrams daily for nonpregnant women.
450 milligrams daily for pregnant women.
350 milligrams daily for men.

Maximum Recommended Dosage

400 milligrams for nonpregnant women. (Although dosages slightly above this are considered safe, medical supervision is recommended when this limit is exceeded.)

Possible Deficiency Symptoms

Irritability, nervousness, muscle weakness, high blood pressure, convulsions, tremors, arrhythmia.

Prevalence of Deficiencies

Surveys indicate that average daily diets contain only 200 to 250 milligrams of magnesium. Deficiencies may be especially widespread in pregnant women. One study of expectant mothers revealed that most got only 60 percent or less of the RDA of magnesium.

Toxic Shock Syndrome Responds to Mineral Replacement

In toxic shock syndrome (TSS), the rare but sometimes fatal disorder found predominantly but not exclusively in menstruating women, doctors know that calcium deficiency is common. What they don't know is what role magnesium plays in this disease.

J. H. Rudick, M.D., of Case Western Reserve University in Cleveland, and a colleague discovered that magnesium depletion may be a little-known finding in TSS—a feature that could contribute to the severity of hypocalcemia (low levels of calcium in the blood) found in TSS patients.

The doctors examined two women with TSS and found low magnesium levels and functional hypoparathyroidism—two conditions known to sometimes accompany one another. "We conclude," Dr. Rudick says, "that life-threatening hypocalcemia in certain magnesium-depleted TSS patients may be averted by magnesium replacement therapy. And it seems reasonable that physicians should consider testing magnesium levels in TSS cases."

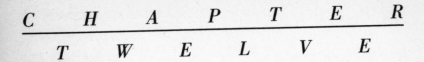
Zinc: The Whole-Body Mineral

It has only been since 1974 that zinc was recognized as essential and given a Recommended Dietary Allowance (RDA) of 15 milligrams daily. But in that short time, this trace mineral has been shown to have a profound influence on the body's ability to grow and to resist disease. Male sexual maturity and fertility depend on adequate zinc. And some researchers think our declining ability to absorb zinc, along with other nutrients, as we age is one reason we become more vulnerable to disease.

So far, researchers have found more than 90 zinc-dependent enzymes in the body—more than those of all the other minerals combined, including iron. Each is involved in a different biochemical reaction. But we need to know only two closely related facts about zinc to understand a good part of its importance.

The Facts about Zinc and Basic Good Health

First, zinc is needed for the body to make protein. Zinc-containing enzymes help to string together the long chains of amino acids that make up each molecule of protein.

Second, every cell's genetic material, its DNA and RNA, is derived from protein.

What this means is that your body needs zinc to make every one of its cells—from the hair on your head to the soles of your feet. Severe deficiencies mean that needed cells may not get made. They also mean that it is more difficult to repair damaged genetic material.

Because cell growth is so dependent on zinc, it's first missed when or where rapid cell growth occurs—in pregnancy, childhood, wound healing and any other situation involving rapidly dividing cells. One of these areas is the immune response.

"Severe zinc deficiency has been shown to cause major abnormalities in the body's immune defense," says Susanna Cunningham-Rundles, Ph.D., at the New York Hospital/Cornell Medical Center in New York City.

One reason for this impact is that any effective immune response involves a massive buildup of the white blood cells that fight bacteria, viruses and cancer. For instance, one type of white blood cell, called a neutrophil, can multiply five times within a few hours after infection sets in. And another kind of white blood cell, called a lymphocyte, can divide and form up to 500 new cells in four days.

"Studies show that if zinc is not present in the quantities needed, this sort of cell proliferation is reduced, and the immune response will be lessened," Dr. Cunningham-Rundles says.

And there are other roles zinc plays in the immune response.

"Zinc is probably essential for the work of thymic hormones," Dr. Cunningham-Rundles says. These hormones, secreted by the thymus gland, are responsible for the development of T-cells, types of lymphocytes central to the fight against viral and bacterial infections.

Zinc will also increase the activity of lymphocytes called natural killer cells, even when there is not an apparent zinc deficiency. Because these cells are able to destroy a virus- or bacteria-invaded cell without the prior sensitization that all other lymphocytes require, they are considered part of the body's first line of defense against disease.

Zinc also seems to interact with vitamin A, a nutrient that seems to have a protective effect against cancer. Certain cells, called epithelial cells, may be particularly dependent on both vitamin A and zinc. These cells cover a surface, such as the skin, or line a cavity, such as the bladder. It's not incidental that these cells also have the most rapid

Zinc, the Thymus and Immunity

We all know that it's our immune system that comes between us and disease. But for some (especially older people and children with Down's syndrome), the system all too often fails. In the past, doctors usually placed the blame on a faulty thymus gland.

Italian researchers have found that a deficiency of zinc (and not the thymus) may be directly responsible for at least part of that failure in these two groups of people. Here's how.

The thymus puts out a hormone called FTS, which is needed for immunity. But this hormone's activity is dependent on zinc. When the researchers measured FTS and zinc levels in these patients, they found both a zinc deficiency and diminished FTS activity.

The researchers think that even marginal zinc deficiencies (which are widespread) may impair FTS activity. Therefore, "careful zinc monitoring should be applied to all patients who show low FTS activity."

turnover of any in the body. Or that throat cancers have been linked with both vitamin A and zinc deficiencies.

One area where epithelial cells are found is in the mammary glands. Michael Bunk, Ph.D., a research scientist at Memorial Sloan-Kettering Cancer Center in New York City, found that mice made zinc deficient also became deficient in vitamin A.

"It's pretty well known that zinc deficiency affects the release of stored vitamin A from the liver," Dr. Bunk says. He thinks there may be a second connection, that a zinc deficiency impairs the uptake of vitamin A by the epithelial cells, putting them at risk for developing cancer or other diseases.

Links with Eating Disorders

Doctors have known for some time that too little zinc can alter the senses of taste and smell. A lack of zinc changes the chemistry of saliva, which directly affects the way things taste in the mouth. Zinc-poor people have trouble tasting sweets, for instance.

But zinc may also affect areas of the brain that receive and process information from taste and smell sensors. And that, in part, has led some researchers to speculate that zinc could influence areas of the brain that control eating and drinking behavior.

"Animal studies seem to indicate that zinc deficiencies could play a role in eating disorders like anorexia and bulimia," says Craig McClain, M.D., associate professor of medicine and director of the Division of Gastroenterology at the University of Kentucky School of Medicine, Lexington. Studies he and his colleagues have done indicate that zinc-deprived rats develop the same bizarre eating habits as teenage girls diagnosed as anorexic, bulimic or bulimirexic, a combination of both disorders. Like the girls, the zinc-deprived rats ate less and less until they were consuming only about a third the normal amount. When they did eat, they tended to pig out, and they also tended to easily regurgitate their food. What's more, when they were subjected to stress (mildly pinched tails), they headed straight for the rat chow! When adequate zinc was added to their diet, the rats' eating behavior returned to normal.

In another study, Dr. McClain found that nine bulimirexic women were extremely low in zinc, even when they were within normal weight ranges and other nutritional signs were normal. "Many of these women's habits—laxative abuse, vomiting, dieting—would definitely put them at risk for a zinc deficiency," Dr. McClain says.

One question is, which comes first, the zinc deficiency or the eating problem? "It's possible that a zinc-poor diet, which wouldn't be all that unusual in teenage girls, could trigger eating problems," Dr. McClain says. "Or the eating problem could be triggered by psychological or social problems."

Can zinc supplements help anorexics break the habit? Perhaps, Dr. McClain says. "That's what we intend to study next. Until results are in with humans, though, about the only recommendation I can give people with eating disorders is to make sure they're getting the RDA of zinc."

Zinc, Alcohol and Obesity

Surprising connections also seem to exist between zinc deficiencies, alcohol abuse and obesity, says Platon Collipp, M.D., former professor of pediatrics at the State University of New York, Stony Brook.

He found that rats fed zinc-deficient diets voluntarily drank much more alcohol than rats fed adequate zinc. (The rats could choose between water and alcohol in their cages.) When they were then given enough zinc, their drinking declined to normal.

"People have been speculating for some time now that food intake can influence drinking behavior. I think zinc is one nutrient that could have a possible effect," says Dr. Collipp. "It would be very interesting to see how or if zinc reduces the craving for alcohol in alcoholics. I haven't been able to do that study, but it should be done. So should a study to see whether zinc supplementation in the children of alcoholics, who may be genetically zinc deficient, reduces their five-times-greater-than-normal chances of becoming alcoholics themselves."

Dr. Collipp also made an interesting discovery that may help some heavyweights. He found that a zinc deficiency is associated with the way the body handles glucose (blood sugar).

Zinc and Vaccinations

Keeping your body's immune function at its best does more than prevent disease from occurring. It's also what helps make you well again when a nasty germ does get in. Either way, it can't do the job alone. That's where zinc comes in.

In one study, scientists from Michigan State University in East Lansing found that without enough zinc, the body may lose its ability to remember what it's been immunized against. The zinc deficiency may actually destroy the so-called immune memory cells, making it virtually impossible to successfully vaccinate against common diseases.

The researchers point out that simply improving the diets of malnourished people may not be enough to restore their immune response to some diseases they've previously been exposed to or vaccinated for. These people may need to be vaccinated after their bodies' nutritional stores of zinc have once again been brought up to optimal levels.

A zinc-dependent enzyme in the liver acts as a kind of railroad switch in glucose metabolism. Called a branch-point enzyme, it's located right at the spot in glucose metabolism where one reaction leads to energy burning and the other to fat storage.

"Studies of rat livers show that when there's not enough zinc to go around, this enzyme becomes inactive," Dr. Collipp says. "The result is that glucose is shunted toward making triglycerides [blood fats] that can be stored in the fatty tissues rather than being burned for energy.

"There are some people who say that everything they eat turns to fat," he says. "Well, those people may be zinc deficient."

Dr. Collipp also thinks there may be psychological connections in zinc's effect on eating and drinking. Zinc-deficient children don't seem to rely on "internal cues" for their behavior, he says. Such children might not be able to discern the difference between feeling hungry and feeling full, for instance.

"Quite a few studies link zinc deficiencies with brain disorders, such as learning problems," Dr. Collipp says. "I think a zinc deficiency may also affect some part of the brain involved in the self-monitoring of the body, a kind of satiation center that lets you know when you've had enough to eat or drink."

Healthy Gums Need Zinc

Zinc deficiency is especially detrimental to the gums. The tissue is loaded with fibrous protein strands, and the thin layer of cells right next to the tooth's root is epithelium, says Henry Mallek, D.M.D., Ph.D., professor at the Georgetown University School of Dentistry in Washington, D.C.

A zinc deficiency doesn't actually *cause* gum disease. Plaque does. But a deficiency makes the gums much less likely to be able to withstand the bacterial assault of plaque that inflames gums and loosens teeth.

"There are many reasons to think that people with gum disease may have zinc deficiencies," Dr. Mallek says. "I've seen people with long-term gum problems who had conventional treatment. Although it helped, the gums were not completely healthy. But when the zinc deficiency was corrected, the gum problems were resolved."

Zinc for Herpes?

Herpes infections—both the cold-sore and the genital kind—have been found to respond to applications of zinc in experimental treatment. Doctors at Hadassah University Hospital in Jerusalem found that herpes simplex sores treated with zinc healed in about 9½ days, compared with an average of 16 days with other forms of treatment. In Swedish studies, continued use of zinc solution after the sores healed prevented a recurrence. Could zinc someday offer hope to genital herpes victims? An animal study by Patrick Tennican, M.D., director of internal medicine, Spokane, and a clinical associate professor at the University of Washington, Seattle, indicates it might, but only if it's used very early in the course of the disease.

Female mice with genital herpes were treated with either a zinc-soaked sponge, a nonmedicated sponge or oral zinc, which was started two days before they were infected. The difference between the topically treated group and the other two groups was great. Thirty-two percent of the untreated group had moderate to severe herpes symptoms by the ninth day after treatment. Only one animal with topical zinc treatment had these symptoms, and for one day only. The mice receiving oral zinc actually had more symptoms than the control group.

Encephalitis, another sign of herpes infection (in mice *only,* not in humans) was greater in the oral zinc and untreated groups. Both had a 40 percent death rate by the 15th day of the experiment, while none of the topically treated mice died. Dr. Tennican thinks the zinc prevented the herpes virus from multiplying by interfering with essential enzyme systems necessary for its replication.

"I'm afraid the problem with genital herpes is that the virus quickly moves away from the site of infection to where no topical agent is going to reach it," Dr. Tennican says. "The idea of using a zinc solution as a kind of 'morning after' treatment is interesting, but the fact is that there is no known topical treatment that has prevented the recurrence of genital herpes."

Zinc and Fertility

There is probably more zinc in seminal fluid than in any other fluid in the body. That finding led urologist Joel L. Marmar, M.D., to wonder if certain male fertility problems might be caused by a zinc deficiency.

He tested some patients in his Cherry Hill, New Jersey, practice. He reports, "Out of our infertile population, 10 to 15 percent have truly low zinc levels." Zinc, he says, has an apparent influence on the swimming ability of sperm, which must be strong enough to reach a woman's fallopian tubes and penetrate the egg for fertilization to take place.

Dr. Marmar isn't sure exactly why it works, but he has had some success using zinc supplements with that small, select group of infertile patients.

Of course, not every malfunction in our body is necessarily the result of a drop in a nutrient stockpile. But new technology, allowing

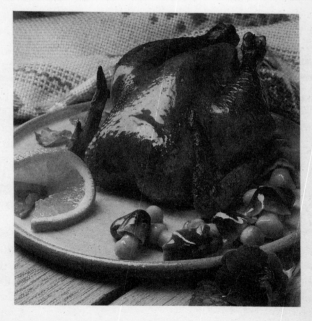

Love chicken livers? Or are you a dark meat fan? Well, whatever part is your favorite, you can be sure that you're also getting a good amount of zinc. Zinc is required by the body for cell growth and development, which makes it a nutritional necessity.

scientists to examine functioning nutrients in living tissue, is helping pinpoint the ones that are.

Zinc for Osteoporosis?

Osteoporosis is a hot topic these days. Increased calcium intake and weight-bearing exercises can help head it off. And it seems zinc might help, too.

Bone metabolism is another area where zinc-dependent enzymes play a role, says Joseph Soares, Ph.D., a professor of nutrition at the University of Maryland, College Park.

In bone calcification in children, the role is clear, Dr. Soares says.

Best Food Sources of Zinc

Food	Portion	Zinc (mg.)
Oysters, raw, meat only	⅓ cup	7.12
Chicken heart, cooked	3 oz.	6.00
Calves' liver, cooked	3 oz.	5.20
Beef liver, braised	3 oz.	5.16
Beef, ground, lean, broiled, medium	3 oz.	4.56
Lamb, lean, cooked	3 oz.	4.20
Pumpkin seeds, roasted	¼ cup	4.20
Tuna, canned in oil, drained	½ cup	4.01
Beef, round, full cut, separable lean only, broiled	3 oz.	3.98
Turkey, dark meat, cooked	3 oz.	3.80
Chicken liver, cooked	3 oz.	3.70
Chicken, dark meat, cooked	3 oz.	2.40
Swiss cheese	2 oz.	2.20
Cashews, dry roasted	¼ cup	1.90
Cheddar cheese	2 oz.	1.80
Sunflower seeds, dry roasted	¼ cup	1.70
Turkey, light meat, cooked	3 oz.	1.70

Zinc is needed to produce a matrix of protein threads onto which the bone-forming calcium is laid. In older people, though, the process is much slower. "Calcium deposition and removal continues into old age, but if more calcium is lost than is deposited, osteoporosis will be the result," Dr. Soares says.

"We'd like to find out if zinc can help to boost calcium deposition in the elderly. It would seem to make sense, but it's a difficult question to answer." Dr. Soares's continuing work will determine the role of supplementation in bone calcification in quail and rats. If it does, he says, "an important new development in the study and control of osteoporosis may be available."

One study by researchers in Turkey showed that victims of

Food	Portion	Zinc (mg.)
Brazil nuts, dried	¼ cup	1.60
Black-eyed peas, cooked	½ cup	1.50
Clams, raw, meat only	3 oz.	1.34
Chick-peas, boiled	½ cup	1.25
Lentils, boiled	½ cup	1.25
Peanuts, all types, dry roasted	¼ cup	1.20
Chicken, light meat, cooked	3 oz.	1.10
Peas, cooked	½ cup	1.00
Filberts, dried	¼ cup	0.70
Tuna, light, canned in water	½ cup	0.70
Oats, regular, cooked	½ cup	0.60

SOURCES: Adapted from
Agriculture Handbook Nos. 8-1, 8-5, 8-8, 8-11, 8-12, 8-13, 8-16 (Washington, D.C.: U.S. Department of Agriculture).
Journal of the American Dietetic Association, April 1975.
McCance and Widdowson's The Composition of Foods, by A. A. Paul and D. A. T. Southgate (New York: Elsevier/North-Holland Biomedical, 1978).

osteoporosis had zinc levels 25 percent lower than those without the disease. "Many older people are getting too little zinc, just as they're getting too little calcium, because of overall poor nutrition," Dr. Soares says. In fact, there's evidence to indicate that zinc intake is below the RDA for other groups as well.

A survey by the Beltsville Human Nutrition Research Center in Maryland found that middle-class adults were getting only about three-fourths of the RDA for zinc, averaging 9.9 milligrams a day. Women fared worse. Their intake was only 57 percent of the 15-milligram requirement.

Make your food choices zinc wise. Oysters are the richest source of zinc. Organ meats and beef are the next-best source. Three ounces of lean beef have nearly four milligrams of zinc. Grains and nuts contain fairly good, but probably less absorbable, amounts. (For a list of other zinc-rich foods, see the table on pages 86 and 87.) In fact, a nutritional survey showed vegetarians on low-calorie diets to be at particular risk for zinc deficiencies. (If you feel you need supplemental zinc, don't take more than 30 milligrams a day without medical supervision.)

Zinc research can only continue to confirm how important it is to get the right amount of this essential trace mineral.